The
Lazy Girl's
Guide to Beauty

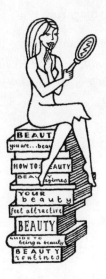

Anita Naik is a freelance writer who has written for *Red*, *New Woman*, *M* magazine, *Cosmopolitan*, *Glamour*, *Now*, and *Men's Health*. She specialises in health, beauty, sex and relationships and is currently the health and advice columnist for *Closer*, and a sex columnist on *More* magazine.

Anita is also the author of:
The Lazy Girl's Guide to Good Health
The Lazy Girl's Guide to Good Sex

The Lazy Girl's Guide to Beauty

Anita Naik

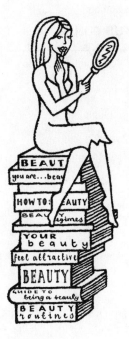

PIATKUS

Visit the Piatkus website!

Piatkus publishes a wide range of bestselling fiction and non-fiction, including books on health, mind, body & spirit, sex, self-help, cookery, biography and the paranormal.

If you want to:

- read descriptions of our popular titles
- buy our books over the internet
- take advantage of our special offers
- enter our monthly competition
- learn more about your favourite Piatkus authors

VISIT OUR WEBSITE AT: www.piatkus.co.uk

Copyright © 2003 by Anita Naik

First published in 2003 by
Judy Piatkus (Publishers) Limited
5 Windmill Street
London W1T 2JA

e-mail: info@piatkus.co.uk

The moral right of the author has been asserted

A catalogue record for this book is available from the British Library

ISBN 0 7499 2399 7

Text design by skeisch and Paul Saunders
Edited by Jan Cutler
Cover and inside illustrations by Nicola Cramp

This book has been printed on paper manufactured with respect for the environment using wood from managed sustainable resources

Printed and bound in Great Britain by
Butler & Tanner Ltd, Frome and London

contents

acknowledgements

With thanks to the many beauty babes who shared their 'being gorgeous' tips, especially Suzanne 'Bambi' Hope, Charlotte Owen-Watson, and Jane Naik. Special gratitude to all the slack beauty babes who inspired this book, especially Emma 'What's shower gel?' Burtenshaw and Denise 'It's really all about hair' Lifton.

introduction

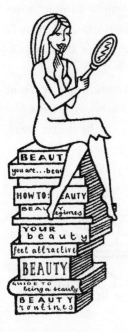

Why this book can help you

Is it just me or is beauty a real bore? Just who is that person who has time to cleanse, tone, moisturise, exfoliate, pluck, pummel, smooth and lovingly nurture their body morning, evening and night? Does she have a life? Better still, I hope she has a job to pay for it all.

If you're currently reading this with mascara smudges etched on to your cheeks, legs as hairy as the New Forest and toothpaste dotted on to your spots, the answer is she's probably not you.

In one way you're to be congratulated for not having succumbed to Botox injections, expensive creams made out of a rhino's bottom and the universal obsession/phobia about cellulite. In fact you're likely to be an au naturel kind of girl and proud of it. However, it's worth noting there is a fine line to be drawn between staying just as nature intended and becoming a part of nature. If your leg hairs are jutting through your 40-denier tights, and your toenails draw blood in the heat of passion, then the chances are you're becoming faintly feral in your approach to looking gorgeous. Which leads to the obvious question: just how long can you get away without injecting some beauty into your beauty routine?

If you've got good genes (look at your older female relations for a clue) you can close this book right now and happily spend your days scoffing at women who have to try harder than you. However, it's worth bearing in mind that a lifetime of indulgence of the non-beauty kind will eventually lead to looks at the dumper end of the looking-good scale.

This means, eat rubbish, refuse to brush your hair, avoid sunscreen and cultivate ET-like hands and by the time you hit the big 40 (not as far away as you might think) you'll resemble an old prune.

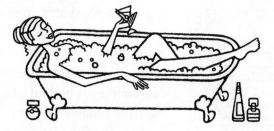

Thankfully though, being beauty-aware doesn't have to mean a complete life overhaul. Or for that matter a trip to your nearest beauty counter and the handing over of your life savings. Lazy beauty costs very little, is actually quite good fun and won't take up your valuable socialising time. Plus, it has less to do with home bikini waxes (remember, I'm talking beauty, not torture), and has more to do with spoiling yourself; a pastime even the laziest girl can understand. After all, down-to-earth beauty is about doing something that works for you. Something that makes you feel and look better, and thankfully it's about more than how to put your eyeliner on straight. It's about taking up a routine that's easy – otherwise, let's face it, you won't do it! Remember, look rough and you'll feel rough, look good and you'll be steeped in a glow of self-confidence. Trust me, it's easier than you think.

chapter 1
Face to face

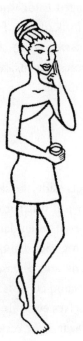

When it comes to beauty, the first and, in some cases, the only place most of us think of doing some work on is our face. Forget hair that resembles barbed-wire netting and toenails that could get a bit-part in a horror movie, the face and skin is where even the laziest beauty babe will attempt to do some DIY. As for those fantastic-looking girls who tell you they never wear make-up, don't bother to moisturise and can't be bothered with a beauty routine, the chances are they're either blessed with great genes, have just had their eighteenth birthday or are lying through their freshly bleached teeth!

The simple fact is everyone has a beauty routine of sorts. It may be more high street than Hollywood but at the end of the day if you do more than wash with soap and clean your teeth (and I am hoping you at least do that) you have a routine. The good news is: for a fabulous face you neither have to spend hours in the bathroom plucking, waxing, smoothing and scrubbing (unless you want to); nor do you need to expand hugely beyond the above soap-and-water scenario, because, despite the adverts that claim otherwise, truck-loads of make-up and expensive creams won't dramatically change the way you look, unless you use a trowel to apply it with (in which case you need a make-up book not a beauty book).

The secret to beautiful, healthy skin is an inside/outside job; roughly translated this means you need to do some internal work as well as external repair. Think of your face as a gorgeous dress: no matter how expensive and good it looks on the outside it won't hang right unless the inside is put together properly and the outside is ironed!

What is skin?

Stupid question really, but, the obvious facts aside, the skin is the body's largest living organ. Not only is it waterproof but also it's amazingly good at repairing itself when damaged, and excellent at setting off warning signs about extremes in temperature, allergic reactions and diseases. The outer sheet is known as the epidermis and consists of billions of layers of cells that renew themselves every three weeks. Old cells drop off at the rate of about 5 per cent a day and make up 90 per cent of household dust. The inner layer is known as the dermis and made up of elastin and collagen, the essential substances you need to have plump, firm skin. It's when this internal layer breaks down (usually with age) that the skin wrinkles and sags.

What's your type?

If you've ever wandered through the beauty section of a department store, at some point you've probably been collared by an assistant who tried to convince you that your 'problem' skin could be easily transformed by handing over your life savings. Beauty tip one: don't be fooled by this jargon. All skin is divided into groups (see below) just as your hair is, and no one type is more problematic than the other. All these skin types do is indicate the kind of skin you have, thanks to your genetic make-up and your lifestyle – i.e. do you smoke, are you a suntan junkie, etc?

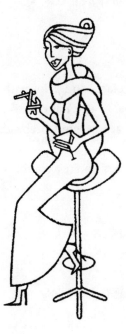

The five types of skin

- Normal
- Combination
- Oily
- Dry
- Sensitive

Normal skin

Contrary to popular thinking, normal skin doesn't mean that you have 100 per cent flawless skin that never has spots or problems. Normal skin is simply skin that isn't dry, oily or sensitive.

Five tips for normal skin

1. Always use a sunscreen.
2. Choose a moisturiser that isn't too rich for your skin type.
3. Avoid strong products that make your skin tingle.
4. Don't overestimate how much abuse your skin can take.
5. Think about a soap-free cleanser.

Combination skin

This isn't skin that peels off in some places and drips with oil in others. It's skin that is categorised by dry, flaky cheeks and an oily T-shaped zone that goes across your forehead and down your nose and chin.

If you have shiny patches in these areas, you're a combination girl.

Five tips for combination skin

1. Use soap with a pH balance, as this is closest to the skin's natural acidity level.
2. Use moisturising cream on your cheeks and apply lightly on your T-zone.

3. Exfoliate only your T-zone area.

4. If you're applying spot treatments, avoid the cheek area.

5. Blot your T-zone before applying make-up.

Oily skin

This is skin which has large pores and looks shiny even when it's not hot. If you're unsure if you're oily or not, place a clean tissue over your face and press down. If the tissue is marked with moisture when you lift it off, you have oily skin. Before you hide under a paper bag it might help to know that a huge plus for people with oily skins is that you will age fantastically well and end up with zero wrinkles.

Five tips for oily skin

1. Don't overwash your face; this just encourages the overproduction of the oil glands.

2. Use lotions rather than creams, as these aren't as heavy on your skin.

3. Don't use toners that make your skin tingle. All this is doing is stripping your skin and will cause it to try to add more moisture by producing more oil.

4. Blot your face with a tissue once you have applied your make-up to stop your foundation from running.

5. Wear sunscreen even if you feel you don't need it.

Dry skin

Skin that looks patchy and red in places is dry. Sometimes the skin will look flaky or chapped. Although this type of skin is prone to wrinkles, the good news is you'll rarely get spots because you have so little oil production going on.

Five tips for dry skin

1. Moisturise more than once a day.
2. Use a high-factor sun cream.
3. Don't use alcohol-based toners and cleansers, as they drink the skin dry.
4. Don't put on powder without moisturising first.
5. Avoid soap on your face.

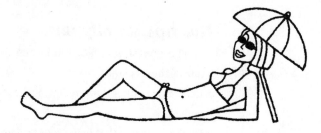

Sensitive skin

Skin that is sensitive reacts quickly to certain soaps, make-up, creams or even fluctuations in temperature. This skin may look as if it's dry, but in reality the skin is irritated and can feel itchy and hot and there may be tiny red lumps on the cheeks.

Five tips for sensitive skin

1. Use unperfumed beauty products.
2. Always patch-test products and wait 24 hrs before applying.
3. Natural doesn't mean better – you can be allergic to anything even if it's made from non-synthetic ingredients.
4. Don't scrub your face with anything harsh.
5. Less is more when it comes to beauty products.

What's what with cleansing, exfoliating, toning and moisturising

Cleansing

Over cleansing means cleaning your face more than once a day and scrubbing/ rubbing/exfoliating and or buffing more than once a week.

Lazy girls rejoice – the number-one complaint beauty therapists have about their clients is that most (if not all) over-cleanse. While it's good news to take off your make-up and wash your face every day, attempting to sandblast your pores in pursuit of cleanliness is a little excessive. Girls who cleanse, wash, scrub, tone and moisturise daily, are not only stripping the skin of natural oils but also emptying their purses for no good reason. At the same time, poor cleansing can leave your skin looking dry and grey and make it more prone to spots, as it allows bacteria to flourish.

To cleanse easily and effectively, all you have to do is:

- Use just one product to remove both your make-up and the day's grime. This can be something as simple as a cold cream, facial soap or a cream-based product.
- Never use a bath soap or heavily perfumed soap on your face. If your skin feels tight, your soap is too strong for your skin.
- The drier your skin the thicker the cleanser you'll need – think creamy textures. The oilier your skin the less creamy the cleanser. Choose a gel-based product or one you can wash off. Normal skins should opt for a runny lotion cleanser that can be wiped off.
- How often you wash your face depends on how dirty it feels. Skin that feels gritty and looks shiny is skin that needs a cleanser.
- Always wash your hands before you start cleansing. Rubbing in cream with hands that haven't been cleaned first is a waste of time.

Exfoliating

When exfoliants first came on the market they were as gritty as pebbledashing and worked on the idea that the harder you rubbed in the sharp bits the smoother your skin would be. These days exfoliating attracts a mixed bag of responses. Many beauty therapists now believe that as the skin naturally renews itself it doesn't need any help in shedding old skin and so exfoliating is a big no-no. Other experts believe simply washing with a face cloth is all the exfoliating you need, as harsher exfoliants can cause more damage to the skin than good.

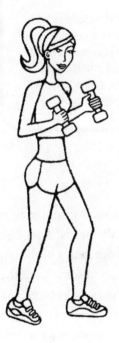

Having said that there are those who still believe slough-ing off dead cells is the only way to have skin like a baby, which is why the market is flooded with various products that insist you scrub away once a week. Whether you choose to use one or not make sure you don't scrub too vigorously. Remember, you're not sanding down a piece of wood, it's your face you're working on. Rub too hard and you'll not only scratch your skin but also leave yourself looking as if you've been sandblasted.

To exfoliate effectively:

- Test the exfoliant on your hand first. If it feels too scratchy and leaves your hand feeling raw, it's too harsh for your face.
- Look for scrubs that have small granules that dissolve when you use them, and rub lightly so you don't cause more harm than good.
- Avoid facial puffs at all cost. If it looks like it could clean your oven you don't want it near your bottom, never mind your face.
- Think natural: if you're really desperate to scrub, think about using oats as an exfoliant.
- Never scrub more than once a week and if you're left with skin that looks red and patchy, your skin's telling you to leave off.

DIY exfoliator

Rather than spending out on an expensive exfoliant, raid your kitchen cupboard and grab some oats. Uncooked oats make a fab exfoliator. All you have to do is take a handful and make it into a paste with some water, and then rub it on to your skin. Don't rub too hard, as the aim is to loosen dead skin cells, not rub your face raw. Then wash off.

Toning

To tone or not to tone, that's the question. Again toning is one of those beauty things no one really needs. Although many claim that toners can shrink your pores and even close them, the truth is they can't. In fact in some cases the wrong toner can actually make your pores looks bigger. As for that fresh-faced feeling, all toner effectively does is wipe off the remainder of your cleanser and replace it with an astringent (usually alcohol-based). Having said that, some people love toners so if you're going to use one here's how:

- Use one that's right for your skin type. If your skin feels tight and tingly afterwards your toner is way too strong for you.
- Smell it before you try it – if the whiff leaves you feeling light-headed, the alcohol level is too high for your skin.

- Don't believe sales people who insist you have to tone as part of a cleansing routine. If your skin looks fine without it, don't be suckered into buying a product.
- Cold water has pretty much the same effect as a toner, so splash some on.
- If you have irritated skin, a gentle toner can help soothe it. Patch-test before use.

Moisturising

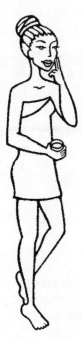

A good face cream is vital for a good complexion, simply because it helps attract water to your skin and helps to hold it there, plus it should boost radiance with ingredients such as added vitamins. However, if you want to feel completely stupid about beauty products then take a look at the shelves that sell face creams. In the space of 30 seconds you'll be swamped with the largest amount of pseudo-scientific babble since you read the back of a cola can. There are creams that say they can protect/soothe/brighten/clear/firm/soften and even take 20 years off you! Some have weird-sounding ingredients like AHAs, others have vitamin C or retinol or are non-comedogenic – or oil-free – the list is endless, and unless you're an expert, you probably buy your product by its packaging or opt for the cheapest cream available. Getting to grips with cream is no easy matter, but basically whatever pot you choose or however much you decide to hand over for it, what you should be looking for is a cream that actually works on you. This means a cream that rubs in easily, does not irritate your skin and does its job effectively so that two hours later your skin is not as parched as the Sahara or shinier than a polished spoon. Apart from thinking about your skin type when choosing a cream consider:

- Your age – different moisturisers are formulated for different types of skin.
- The environment you work in – is it dry and heavily air-conditioned? If so, go for a cream that will moisturise, rather than a lotion. Do you work outside a lot? If so, buy a product that incorporates a skin protector to protect you from the harsh elements.
- How lazy you are about your skin – if you know you're not going to put eye cream, night cream or sunscreen on as well, buy a cream you can use for everything.

tip

All face creams are not created equal. However, if it works for you, keep using it. Everyone's skin is different. If an expensive cream works for your best friend, it doesn't necessarily mean it will work for you.

What's what with face-cream ingredients

- AHAs, also known as alpha hydroxy acids, are fruit acids usually derived from natural products, which work by supposedly boosting the exfoliating process. They work well on normal and combination skins but are too harsh for dry and sensitive skins.
- Ceramides are said to work on a cell level and help the skin by supporting the structure and trapping moisture. They are usually found in creams for older women.

- Liposomes apparently go further into the outer layer of the skin than any other type of cream, allowing your moisturiser to go deeper, giving you softer skin.
- Antioxidants are the A, C and E vitamins that help combat the damage from free radicals, such as pollution, smoke and the sun, and so keep your skin young-looking. Though they're now found in plenty of creams, it's still best to get your daily dosage from your food.
- Retinol (better known as vitamin A), which helps maintain the firmness of the skin by boosting collagen production.

myth

Haemorrhoid cream is a fab anti-ageing facelift cream. Untrue. Haemorrhoid creams contain a variety of chemicals that are designed to relieve anal itching and pain, and reduce inflammation. While it's possible that some of the ingredients can tighten skin, apply it to your face and you could have a minor cosmetic disaster. After all it doesn't take a genius to know what's good for the bum isn't good for the face.

Protecting your skin

Want to avoid looking like a wizened 60-year-old when you're 40? Then help yourself by *not sun-worshipping* and that includes tanning beds too. If you insist of sitting in the sun with zero protection on, no amount of expensive face creams, facials, make-up and healthy food will keep your face looking young and beautiful. If you don't believe me, check out one of the endless studies which show that 95 per cent of all skin ageing is down to sun damage. Of course, the reality is 75 per cent of people won't wear sunscreen, because they still think a tan looks healthy, and one in five of us won't wear protection because it's just 'too much hassle'.

Among this figure are the millions of people who still regularly top up their tans with a sunbed, even though a sunbed emits radiation similar to that of the midday summer sun: just ten minutes can be as powerful as a whole day in the sun.

The problem with UVA and UVB sunrays is they damage your skin on an external and internal level leaving you prone to wrinkles, liver spots and a whole variety of health worries including skin cancer. While we all know the only safe tan comes out of a bottle, you can reduce the risks to your face and avoid being one of the millions of new cases of skin cancer a year by:

- Not bingeing on sunlight. Baking yourself over a weekend causes maximum damage to your skin cells even if you stay out of the sun for the rest of the summer.
- Always wearing a sunscreen in the sun and on cloudy summer days with a minimum protection factor of no less than SPF 15.

Reapply every two hours and don't be fooled into thinking you can decrease the protection factor as the time goes on. A tanned face does not become resilient to ultraviolet rays.

- Wearing sunscreen even if you're under a shaded umbrella, as pavement, sand and water all reflect 85 per cent of the sun's rays.
- Thinking about what you're doing in the sun. If you're going to go swimming and/or play sport, reapply more frequently and go for a higher factor, as you'll sweat more and be more exposed.
- Making sure you use enough. It's tempting to sparsely apply your sunscreen but you need a fair-sized dollop for each area of your body, and one equal to the size of a 50 pence piece for your face.

Troubleshooting in the sun

You've burnt your face

Don't fool yourself that a tan makes you look healthy. It may do you wonders now, but in 10 years you'll look more like a dried prune.

Cool yourself down. Soak the burnt area in cold water or place a cold flannel over it for ten minutes at least. Then apply a natural soothing gel or cream such as aloe vera or calendula and drink plenty of water. After you've soothed it, keep it covered in the sun by wearing a hat, and apply a total sunblock to the area to stop further damage.

A rash appears in the heat

Polymorphic light eruption (PLE) is a reaction to UV radiation from the sun, and it affects 15 per cent of people.

It can be soothed by moving out of the sun and into a cool room, and by applying a cold compress. To avoid PLE, use high-protection sun factors, and those containing zinc oxide, which is a chemical block that literally shields the skin.

Sandpaper lips

Lips have zero protection against the sun simply because the skin here is at its thinnest. Lipstick can add an SPF of around 4, which is even more reason to apply a lip balm with SPF 15 and keep applying it after swimming, and after drinking and eating.

Your make-up is sliding off your face

Sunscreens take time to sink in and so should be applied at least 40 minutes before you put your slap on. Sunblocks on the other hand are meant to lie on your skin to form a barrier and should not be rubbed in until they disappear. For best results, apply make-up and then pat sunblock over the top. Use a gel, if you don't want to ruin your look.

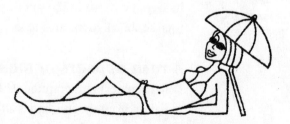

You've been attacked by a horde of bloodthirsty mosquitoes

Not quite the look you were hoping for on your face. If your bites have swollen up, and remained itchy the chances are you are allergic to the nasty critters. To help ease your discomfort think about dabbing the bites with calamine (the pink stuff your mum once put on your chickenpox) and/or an antiseptic cream. Then add a few drops of citronella essential oil to your sunscreen, as this is a natural insect repellent.

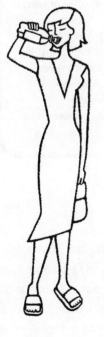

The hydration factor aka drink more water

Research from the Natural Water Information Service in the UK shows one in five people consume too little water throughout the day. The current recommendation is at least 1.5 litres (2½ pints or about 8–10 glasses), which means most of us suffer from borderline dehydration. This is bad news for our skin, because the body is about 70 per cent water, and 35 per cent of that is found in the skin, which means when you're dehydrated the first thing the body does is grab moisture from the skin.

By comparison, drinking the right amount of water not only hydrates the skin but also flushes through the kidneys, which then gets rid of toxins and therefore makes the skin appear healthier.

Unsure if you need more water? Then look at your urine. The darker the colour the more dehydrated you are, and the more water you need to drink. If the thought of guzzling ten glasses a day is too much for you, think of it as half a glass of water every half an hour, and you'll easily hit your quota.

For better skin

- Drink two extra glasses of water for every coffee or glass of wine you drink.
- Keep alcohol to a minimum – for every 1 ml (less than ¼ teaspoon) of alcohol drunk, 10 ml (2 teaspoons) is lost in urine and fluids. Alcohol also acts as a diuretic in your system, which means it tricks your body into over-urinating, leading to an exaggerated fluid loss.
- On average opt for a 250 ml (8 fl oz) glass of water every hour.

Luscious lips

OK, you may have knocked your skin and face into shape, but don't forget your lips, especially if you're planning on getting some kissing action in someday soon. Many of us tend to neglect our lips because on the whole they look pretty juicy compared to the rest of our face. However, if

you want them to stay that way here's what you should
be doing:

- Use a balm at least once a week. These are designed to protect,
  soothe and seal the lips helping them to remain moist and
  supple. Most balms are made of the same fatty substances so
  you don't have to go expensive to get the right moisture. In fact
  good old Vaseline will do just fine and if you want it to look like
  lip gloss just add a bit of your lipstick to the mix.
- Wear a protective balm with an SPF of at least 15 in the summer
  and in extreme weather. Lips lack melanin – the body's natural
  protection against the sun and elements; this means they will
  burn easily in the sun and chap in the wind.
- Watch out for cold sores. These unsightly blisters are caused by
  the herpes simplex virus and are often triggered by the sun's UV
  rays. Help avoid them by never kissing someone who has one
  (they spread like wildfire) and by dabbing on a dot of tea tree oil
  the second you feel a tingle. For a stronger response try an over-
  the-counter product from the pharmacist, such as Zovirax. To
  disguise a cold sore, try some concealer applied with a cotton
  bud (but not if it's open and weeping).
- Plump your lips. It's not your imagination; as you get older
  the lips get thinner due to the production of collagen slowing
  down. To plump your lips (see Chapter 4, too) and keep them
  sexy, there are a variety of products you can buy. Look for
  lip-enhancing gels, which work by stimulating blood flow.

myth

You can get addicted to lip balm. Untrue. While you might get used to the feel of moist lips and therefore not want to be without your balm, there's no ingredient within these products that will cause you to get a chemical dependency upon the product.

Eye eye!

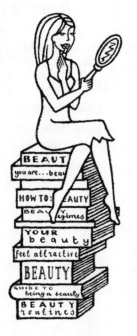

Perhaps your biggest asset on the beauty front is your eyes. Not only do they sparkle without any added beauty trick but also when it comes to sexual attraction they're the first port of call on any sensible man's list. To enhance their beauty status all you need do is the same old thing you've been doing since you were 15 years old: lash mascara over your eyelashes and add colour to your lids. If you're especially lazy, you can even get away with just using Vaseline, which not only lengthens your eyelashes but also gives your lids a natural sparkly sheen.

The only real problem with eyes is the area of skin that surrounds them. This is made up of delicate skin that is prone to fine lines and wrinkles. Get too stressed, squint (because you're too vain to get glasses), refuse to wear sunglasses in the sun and hang about in smoky environments and this area will get puffy, lined and/or look dark and dreary in no time.

To help this area, all you need to do is protect your eyes from environmental pollution. Some experts suggest a daily eye cream, others a more gentle normal cream (patch-test the area before you slap anything on) but if you're sensible you can get away with a pair of polarised sunglasses – these give the most protection from sunlight.

Eye troubleshooting

Dry, red eyes

You need more vitamin A. Lack of this vitamin can cause the eyes' natural secretions to dry up making them red and painful. Beta-carotene, found in foods rich in vitamin A, such as carrots and apricots, is a powerful antioxidant and will help protect the eyes from smoky environments and sunlight. If you're going to take vitamin A in supplement form, be sure it's in a multivitamin and follow the dosage instructions.

Red eyes and styes

These occur when the tear ducts get blocked and the eyelash follicle gets blocked and then infected. Vitamin C (found in citrus fruits and spinach) helps avoid this, as it boosts the immune system and helps reduce inflammation.

tip

When taking off your eye make up be gentle with the skin under your eyes. Avoid dragging it down to your chin or across to your ears, unless you want bags.

Dark circles

These can be hereditary but tend to become more noticeable as you age and your skin loses its natural firmness. Lack of sleep also encourages this appearance as blood rushes into the blood vessels causing that shadowy look. The best cure is simply regular sleep. To help aid this try drinking camomile tea. Apart from encouraging good sleep, it helps reduce facial tension and therefore reduces the formation of dark circles.

Bags under your eyes

While nothing can get rid of bags for good (apart from plastic surgery) you can help reduce that puffy look with one of the following: cucumber slices, cold teabags and ice wrapped in a flannel. For more permanent solutions cut down on salt, as this can also cause bags to inflate.

Spot coverage

Did you imagine you'd be able to chuck out your spot creams the second you hit your eighteenth birthday? Well, if you did you're not alone. Sadly, though, our hormones have other ideas, which is why so many of us are hit by premenstrual zits. A spot usually occurs because the sebaceous glands, which are responsible for producing sebum (oil) for the skin, go into overproduction and clog up a skin pore, leaving the pore to become inflamed with bacteria. If your spots aren't linked to your periods, then they could be the result of your make-up or face cream. Go for a non-comedogenic cream, which means it won't block your pores. Other ingredients that can cause a spot flare-up on your face include:

- Mineral oils, like Vaseline, which lie on the skin and can block pores.
- Lanolin, which is found in lots of creams and sunscreens.

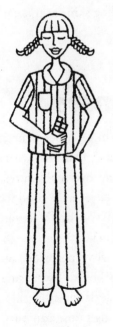

Spot dos and don'ts

Do eat chocolate and chips

Contrary to popular belief, spots are not caused by eating chocolate and junk food. People only think they're linked because we usually crave sweet things when we're premenstrual – a time when our hormones are naturally surging and giving us spots.

Do go for a make-up cover-up

Especially if you have a hot date, try to keep the spot dry before you pile on the foundation and avoid covering a weeping pustule.

Don't make it into a beauty spot

Really, believe me, this won't fool anyone!

Do pick it

But only if it has come to the surface (see below).

Don't try to scrub it off your face

Over-cleansing and scrubbing will just encourage more oil production and may break the spot open and cause scarring.

Do try a spot cream

You're never too old to use a spot zapper, but make sure it hits just the spot and not the surrounding skin (as this can damage this area).

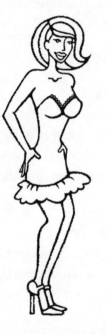

Medicated responses

If you're prone to less than flawless skin on a permanent basis, a medicated response may be better than just wishing your spots away. While there are no overnight cures, over-the-counter products can help. Give each product you use an eight-week chance, and if you don't see an improvement after that, try something new.

Look for products containing benzoyl peroxide, an oxidising agent that will act against blackheads by causing your skin to peel and reducing bacteria on the skin. However, watch how much you use: a high dose can burn *myth*

Apply toothpaste to zap a zit. Untrue. It might help dry them up, but at the same time toothpaste is more likely to do harm than good. If it's great at cleaning your teeth it's likely to irritate your skin and leave red sore patches and flaking skin – often worse than a spot.

the skin. Or try a product with azelaic acid; this unblocks clogged-up hair follicles and also loosens blackheads.

If over-the-counter products don't work for you, see your doctor for oral antibiotics or even the pill (certain brands can help with acne). Or ask for a referral to a dermatologist who can provide you with Roaccutane (available only on prescription), a powerful drug that helps dry up excess oil, stop sebum production and reduce scarring.

Although not clinically proven, there is anecdotal evidence to suggest that natural products can help you get a clear complexion. Try:

Spirulina: a blue/green algae that can be used as a mask or taken orally. It contains all eight amino acids and it's these that are said to work against spots.

Zinc: 30 mg a day taken as a supplement is said to help keep your skin clear.

Omega 3 and 6 fatty acids: found in nuts and fish. These can help create anti-inflammatory substances in the body.

Tea tree oil or lavender oil: natural antiseptic oils that can be dabbed on to the affected area.

Lazy girl's guide to squeezing

When a girl's gotta squeeze, a girl's gotta squeeze ...

Step one: start by washing your hands and under your nails with soap; you don't want to spread more bacteria to your face.

Step two: don't use your fingernails unless you want track marks on your skin. Instead use two tissues and the sides of your fingers against the sides of the spots.

Step three: don't squeeze inwards, but pull the skin apart between the sides of your fingers, away from the centre of the spot. If the spot's ready to be squeezed this will work with little effort.

Step four: if that doesn't work, squeeze inwards to create pressure.

Step five: squeeze to release the head, but don't squeeze until the spot bleeds, as this leads to skin bruising.

Step six: the area will be left sore and swollen so to calm it down and help it dry out dab tea tree oil (a natural antiseptic) on to it and don't apply make-up for at least an hour.

A *word about Rosacea*

Rosacea is a chronic acne-like condition that affects one in 100 people usually with fair skin. Symptoms include sporadic flushing on the cheeks, nose, chin and/or forehead accompanied by bumps, pimples and small pustules. In some cases the nose may even become red and swollen. It can't be cured but it can be controlled. There are several triggers that make Rosacea worse:

- Alcohol
- Coffee
- Tea
- Hot spicy foods
- Cheese
- The sun
- Stress

While it can be camouflaged with make-up, your doctor can also prescribe antibiotics to help clear it up.

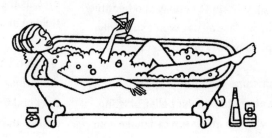

20 ways to fabulous skin

1 Don't rely on your make-up for sun protection

While some daily moisturisers and foundations have SPFs, most will not protect you from the sun in the same way that sunscreen will. Make-up with SPF is designed for light sun exposure only, such as walking to the shops or when you're out at lunch.

2 You can sleep in your make-up

Sleeping with a full face of make-up isn't the huge beauty crime make-up gurus make it out to be. While it's not great for your sheets or for that first morning look in the bathroom mirror, the make-up that quite happily and healthily sat on your face all day won't suddenly turn into a beauty villain over night.

3 Sunshine won't blitz spots

Contrary to popular belief, blasting spots with too much sun can make your skin worse as it increases oil and skin cell production. Help yourself by protecting spotty areas with an oil-free sun product that will stop you from burning and still allow your spots to heal.

4 Ask for beauty samples

Make-up counters always come stocked with a variety of sample-sized creams so before you cough up for anything ask for a trial size so you can see if it works for you. This way you can not only have handy travel-sized beauty products but also (and more importantly) you won't be wasting your money on cream that you'll end up slapping on your bottom.

5 Use an extra pillow

This prevents waking up with puffy eyes, as the angle of your head allows fluid to drain downwards.

6 Don't believe what you read

Simple, but true: if a product sounds too good to be true – it is. There are no creams that can get rid of wrinkles, stop the ageing process or change your complexion overnight.

7 Avoid chapped lips

By drinking more and keeping them well moisturised. The lips dry out because they hold no oil glands to keep them moist and so need water to transport nutrients to the cells and balm to keep them soft.

8 Rub it to make it go further

If you're about to apply any cream, take a smaller dollop than usual and then rub it between your palms first to warm it up and help it spread more easily across your skin.

9 Moisturise on damp skin

Most moisturisers work better if you apply them to damp skin as they help trap moisture and sink in faster.

10 Utilise your kitchen products

Stuck for products to put on your face? Then raid your kitchen cupboards. Oats work well with water as a facial mask or exfoliator. Cucumber slices and cold teabags placed over the eyes can help hydrate skin and reduce puffiness, as they constrict the blood vessels, whereas yoghurt can help soothe sunburn.

11 Change your beauty regime as you age

If you're still doing the same things to your face as you were at 15 years old, it's time to give your make-up bag an overhaul. Oil production starts to slow at 25, and hormonal shifts around pregnancy will affect the way your skin looks and what you'll need to do to it.

12 Chuck out old make-up

While make-up rarely comes with use by dates, nothing lasts forever. Ditch lipsticks dating back five years, foundation from last Christmas and sunscreen for two years ago.

13 Listen to your senses

Cream that smells strange and feels lumpy, or lipsticks that leave a tingle on your lips have gone off so don't use them.

14 Drink tap water

Obviously only if you're in a country where it's tested to high standards. If not opt for purified water (boiled water) or bottled water.

15 Close your pores

Run an ice cube over your pores before applying make-up to help them shrink.

16 Don't stress about night cream

Most top beauty experts, such as the Dr Hauschka French range and Eve Lom, now believe night creams are not essential. If you want to use something at night, just apply your usual moisturiser but remember to do it 30 minutes before you go to bed so it doesn't rub off.

17 Do some aerobic exercise

It's a guaranteed way to keep your skin looking firm, young and fresh. This is because aerobic exercise – running, walking, cycling and swimming – boosts the heart rate and stimulates circulation in the skin.

18 Have more sex

After the age of 25 you will lose, on average, half a pound of muscle every year, and this will be replaced by fat, especially on your face and neck, if you don't do something. Regular sex will help keep things firm, and increase your breathing capacity, which in turn will bring more oxygen to the skin.

19 Let your skin breathe

Your face is like any other part of your body: sometimes it just needs to be naked and free. Try to let it breathe (the skin directly absorbs small amounts of oxygen) by taking off your make-up and leaving it cream-free for a couple of hours a day.

20 Smile more

The muscular contractions it takes to smile are akin to putting your facial muscles through a 45-minute step class. Smile more often (or kiss as this also uses 34 facial muscles) and you won't end up with cheeks on your chest.

chapter 2

Hands, feet, teeth and hairy endeavours

Bad hair, brittle nails, frightening teeth and over-zealous body hair – who hasn't suffered one or more (or all) of these beauty disasters at one time or another? Luckily help is at hand, and you don't need a pair of garden shears or a beautician wielding a vat of wax to help you keep it under control.

Of course, there's the question of why you should bother. And you don't have to, especially, if you want to be seen as more feral than fair. On the other hand, with very little effort and a minimum budget you could transform your wild look in a few easy steps.

Hand and nail care

Nails are made of a brittle fibrous material called keratin. For strong and healthy nail growth – about 3 mm (1/8 inch) per month – you need plenty of B vitamins and zinc. What you don't need is nasty chipped-off nail varnish (screams 'slapper'), chewed-down nails with bleeding cuticles (shouts 'nervous wreck') or talons the length of your nose (it's so 1980s darling!).

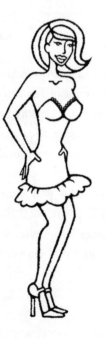

For healthy nails, bear in mind what you're working with. While the part of the nail on show is made up of keratin and is dead, the underlying nail bed is full of blood vessels, which should bring a pink glow to your nails. At the edges of the nail, the skin overlaps and this is known as the cuticle. Cutting this area, chewing it down or trying to push it back during a manicure is not the best idea, as the cuticle protects the nail bed from germs and fungal infections. Like your hair and skin, your nails will need very little beauty work and will already look shiny with a smooth surface, if you're in good health. If not, they will probably be crumbly and quick to snap. Here's how to boost their beauty potential.

The five-minute manicure

- **Step one:** trim nails (don't bite them off or rip them) to the length you want and then file them into shape with a buffer (this also shines the nail).

- **Step two:** rub oil or cream into the cuticles and then soak in warm water for 1 minute. Massage your hands as you exfoliate and rinse.

- **Step three:** dry and then gently push cuticles back with an orange stick and clean under the nails with varnish remover and over the tops of nails to get rid of any old polish. Massage on hand cream.

- **Step four:** now apply a base coat of polish if you're going for a colour and then two coats of polish.

- **Step five:** lie back on the sofa and allow at least two minutes for the polish to dry.

Nail troubleshooting

Problem: split, flaking nails.

Reason: constantly dipping your hands and nails into strong soaps can cause flaking and splitting. This is because the detergent (which you probably use to wash grease off your plates) wears down the surface of the nail, stripping the keratin.

Help yourself by: wearing rubber gloves when you wash up.

Problem: brittle nails.

Reason: bad diet.

Help yourself by: eating more dairy products, spinach, carrots, dried apricots and oily fish and seafood. This will add iron, vitamin A, vitamin B6, and zinc to your body – essential for strong nails. Also make sure you cut your nails instead of biting them off as this makes them prone to flaking.

Problem: yellow nails.

Reason: nail varnish overdose.

Help yourself by: always removing your nail varnish and washing the nails with soapy water before reapplying. Then always use a base coat to protect the nail plate from staining.

Problem: nails with white spots.

Reason: not a sign of a lack of calcium but either a mild trauma (such as a knock) to the nail plate as the nail was growing or a sign of a zinc deficiency.

Keep your nails beautiful

By:
- Regularly filing them into shape. Avoid a metal file, as this is often too strong for the nail.
- Use acetone-free nail varnish, which won't dry out the nail and leave it flaking.
- Rub moisturising cream into the hands and nails daily.
- Give yourself a break from false nails (at least every two weeks).
- Use a nailbrush to clean under the nail and whiten the tip.
- Don't forget to protect your hands in the sun.
- For a real boost, use a face mask on your hands once a week.
- Massage your hands and fingers to improve circulation – move from the wrist all the way up the length of one finger, and repeat.

Give your nails a rest from nail varnish especially if you have discoloration. To make yellow nails look healthy soak in lemon juice for five minutes, moisturise and always use a base coat to protect the surface of the nail.

Help yourself by: eating more pulses, seafood, red meat and pumpkin seeds to increase zinc levels in your diet.

Problem: hangnails.

Reason: these are caused by lack of folic acid and a vitamin C deficiency.

Help yourself by: eating at least four to five servings of fruit and green leafy vegetables a day.

Problem: pale nail beds.

Reason: pale or bluish nail beds are a sign of anaemia and iron deficiency.

Help yourself by: increasing your intake of meat, sardines and cereal.

Looking after your feet

We apparently walk an amazing 70,000 miles in a lifetime, and most lazy girls do it in the most inappropriate of shoes. This means that on the beauty front most of us have feet that could not only do with a pedicure but also some industrial sandblasting, too. Take a look at your feet (if you can bear to). Are your toenails in need of filing, do you have corns, itchy patches, red bumps and hard skin on the soles of your feet? Would your feet get a bit-part in a horror movie? If so here are ten areas where you're going wrong:

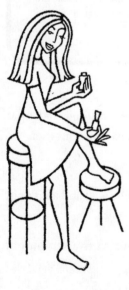

1. You squeeze your feet into shoes that are too tight in the width.
2. You wear trainers all the time.
3. You never file your toenails after cutting them.
4. You don't remove old nail varnish before slapping on a new coat.
5. You never moisturise the soles of your feet.

6. You don't protect them from the sun.

7. Comfort and shoes don't go hand in hand for you.

8. You wear very high shoes all the time.

9. You don't let your feet breathe.

10. You wear stockings and tights all the time.

Festering feet is the main result of all the above, along with a collection of corns, bunions, athlete's foot, achy feet and an abundance of dead skin. Would you let your face get into this state? I think not. Of course, it's easy to forget about feet in winter because, let's face it, they spend much of their lives hidden away. However, come the summer, there's nothing sexy about scratchy, claw-like feet being crammed into a pair of sex-kitten sandals when you're partying! Here's how to treat your feet more kindly all year round:

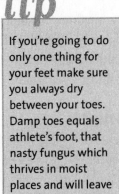

tip

If you're going to do only one thing for your feet make sure you always dry between your toes. Damp toes equals athlete's foot, that nasty fungus which thrives in moist places and will leave your feet itchy and peeling for weeks.

See a chiropodist

Not a pedicurist, who will just basically wash your feet and paint your nails, but a trained foot expert, who will cut and trim your nails, scrape off hard skin and tell you where you're going wrong with your foot care.

Cut your nails properly

This means straight across. Don't follow the curve of the toe or else you're asking for ingrown toenails – where the nail starts pressing into the skin around your toes causing pain and discomfort when you walk.

Use a pumice stone

This volcanic rock (or you can use a synthetic version) helps slough off layers of dead skin that collect on the ball of the foot – where high shoes exert the most pressure – and on the heel. Use in the bath. Look for dry, white skin.

Moisturise your feet every night

Use a strong cream with lanolin, as this is the most moisturising. Rub in and then put cotton socks on. It will give you soft baby feet in no time.

Soak your feet once a day

It's not only relaxing but also helps ease achy feet muscles and makes it easy to massage afterwards.

Massage once a day

This improves circulation and thereby improves the look of your feet. Start at the base of your foot and, using your thumbs, massage the arch, toes and sole of your feet, moving towards the ankle and then your calves.

Varnish properly

This means taking off your old stuff at least once a week and washing the nails with soapy water before reapplying.

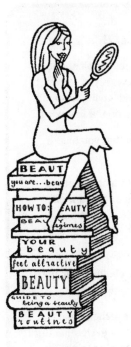

Treat your nasty bits

Athlete's foot is a virulent fungal infection, but it can be treated simply and easily by buying an over-the-counter antifungal treatment or rubbing in tea tree oil. Be sure to dry between each toe, as it's moist conditions that cause the growth of bacteria and allow athlete's foot spores to take hold.

Fungal nail infections are harder to zap, as the nail is impervious to nail paint. More often than not a trip to your doctor for antifungal tablets is your best bet (keep taking them as it takes a while to clear up).

Corns and calluses not only look unsightly but also keep building up, causing pressure on the sides of your feet.

Foot odour affects over 50 per cent of men and 40 per cent of women. This is because we all have 250,000 sweat glands in our feet, and the moist, humid conditions of our shoes make that area the perfect breeding ground for bacteria. Together sweat and bacteria make up a rather foul combination. To help with smelly feet, wash feet every day and dry with a cornflour-based talc. This helps absorb sweat. Let feet breathe once a day with no shoes or socks. Don't wear the same pair of shoes all day every day.

The five-minute pedicure

Unlike a trip to the chiropodist, pedicures are all about beautifying your toes, and the good news is you can do it to yourself in five easy minutes. To avoid having to spend hours on them each month, ensure you do the following:

- **Step one:** moisturise and exfoliate so that you have a good base to work from.

- **Step two:** strip off existing polish with a non-acetone remover (this will stop the nail drying out) and sneak around edges and under the nail with a cotton bud dipped in remover.

- **Step three:** file your nails in one direction into a roundish shape, but avoid the sides or else you could end up with ingrown toenails.

- **Step four:** if your toes are crammed together, separate with cotton wool so they don't rub on to each other until dry. Now apply a base coat to avoid staining the nail.

- **Step five:** if you're right-handed, apply your nail varnish on both toes from right to left, i.e. on the right foot work from the big toe to the little toe/on the left foot work from the little toe to the big toe. This reduces the risk of smudging the nail varnish. Apply the colour in thin, even coats that go up and down the nail, not across, up and over the nail. Keep your arm steady; help yourself by sitting on the floor and leaning towards your toes with your knees bent.

- **Step six:** tidy up any messy edges with a cotton bud. Now wriggle them about as they dry – it's good for your circulation.

Teeth

According to research, when you meet someone, the second place they look at after your eyes is your teeth. If you're displaying a white, uniform smile you'll give the impression of beauty and youth but grin with grubby, stained, irregular ones and he'll be running for the door.

Bearing in mind the above it's hardly surprising that cosmetic dentistry is the one area that's literally booming both with new treatments and new clients. Got teething problems? Here's how to get them fixed.

Bleaching or teeth whitening

Desperate to undo the effects of too much coffee, red wine and Indian takeaways? Well join the queue. The most popular beauty treatment of the moment is teeth-whitening. Here's how to do it:

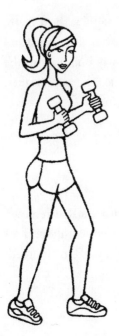

- See your dentist. In surgery, treatment involves painting a gel on to the teeth, which eventually changes the structure of the teeth and makes them whiter. Patients are also given a mouth plate with gel to use at night. The in-surgery technique takes 40 minutes, while the nightly technique takes about two weeks.

- Whitening toothpaste can help maintain the brightness after seeing your dentist, but on its own cannot do more than remove surface stains.
- Avoid DIY bleaching kits. These can be dangerous, as many allow the gel to touch the gums, which can cause irritation problems on the gum.
- Is it painful? No.

Cosmetic contouring

What does it do? This process helps lengthen short teeth, and shorten longer teeth, and also even out chips and fractures in teeth. It's achieved by slowly building up the enamel of a tooth with bonding material. The tooth is then rebuilt and shaped into its original form.

- How long does it take? An hour per tooth.
- Is it painful? No.

Microabrasion

What does it do? This is a polishing process that removes small stains on teeth. A purple glazed compound of hydrochloric acid and pumice is rubbed on to the teeth and then polished off.

- How long does it take? Twenty minutes.
- Is it painful? No.

Porcelain inlays

What do they do? This is the most popular cosmetic dentistry treatment next to bleaching. An inlay is basically a porcelain filling which is made in a laboratory to the exact measurements of your teeth. Unlike a white filling, it is bonded whole and not filled into the teeth in layers. It is tooth-coloured and responds in the mouth like a normal tooth, which means it's kinder to the opposite teeth and longer-lasting.

- How long does it take? Two sessions.
- Is it painful? No.

Veneers

What do they do? If you have a tooth that is damaged or very discoloured, a veneer rather like that of a false nail can be bonded to its surface. Veneers are pre-formed porcelain coverings that are made in a laboratory after an impression is taken of your tooth. The dentist attaches it by shaving 1.5 mm ($\frac{1}{16}$ inch) from the front of your existing tooth and then bonding the veneer on. This is a conservative way of improving the tooth without having to file the tooth down into a stump for a crown.

- How long does it take? Two sessions.
- Is it painful? No.

tip

If you are going to have your teeth bleached (either at the dentist or with a home kit) remember for the first six weeks to avoid foods and drink that may stain your teeth such as red wine, curries, and sugar-based colas.

White fillings

What do they do? Replaces the old silver amalgam fillings. An old filling is taken out of the existing tooth, and a white filling is pasted in. While white fillings are effective and long-lasting, they do not work well in deep fillings.

- How long does it take? Twenty minutes.
- Is it painful? No.

Hair — what to do with it

Have a look at a strand of your hair. Pretty dull isn't it? Well, despite its appearance it's actually a marvel of engineering. We all have around 100,000 hairs on our head, and inside each strand is a mixture of protein, water and lipids (basically fats). On the outside is a protective layer known as the cuticle, which is the part of your hair that appears shiny when healthy and split and flat when it's damaged or when you're ill.

The part of your hair that is alive is the root at the follicle; this is where new hair emerges. The hair we see is essentially dead, and while you can improve its look with products, for healthy glossy-looking hair you need to keep the follicle and root healthy from within (see How To Have Fabulous Hair).

To test your hair's current health:

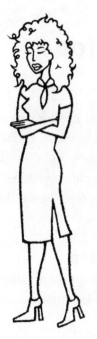

Stretch it when it's wet: healthy hair should stretch about a third of its length before it breaks. To test, pull out a strand from the root and, holding an end with each finger, pull (gently). If it snaps instantly, your hair is damaged or you're lacking in nutrients, which is usually the result of too much partying and junk food.

Look at the ends: split ends are not just a sign you need your hair cut, but also that the hair is dehydrated and has lost moisture and protein. Are you consistently hung over? This will adversely affect the condition of your hair. Do you drink eight glasses of water a day? Have you been protecting your hair with a hat or sunscreen in the sun? All these will have a positive effect.

Sweep your floor: while losing hair is normal (we lose about 100 a day quite naturally) and some hair types lose more hair than others, hair that clogs up your plugholes to the point that you end up with a daily handful of the stuff, or hair that comes out in clumps when you run your hands through it, indicates that all is not well with your internal health. Also, if the fallen hairs are not strands but bits or your hair is falling out more than is normal for you (check your bathroom floor for evidence) your hair is damaged.

Ask yourself — is it limp, lank or luscious?: limp, lank hair that needs a ton of product and hairspray to stay upright is not healthy hair. Whatever your hair type, hair should be bouncy, luscious to touch and able to hold a style for longer than an hour. If not, you've either got product overload, i.e. you're not rinsing your hair properly after washing, or your scalp is too greasy or too dry because of lifestyle issues such as diet, fitness and stress.

How to have fabulous hair

There's no big secret to wonderful hair – as a major part of your body, hair generally responds to the same good stimuli as the rest of your body. Eat well, sleep right, drink enough water and exercise and you, too, can have supermodel hair. If you've got no time for that, here's the shortcut version:

Step one: eat hair-friendly food

Foods that will nourish your hair (if you eat them rather than rub them on) and help give you a shiny, bouncy look are:

- Foods that are rich in omega 3 and 6 essential fatty acids (EFAs). A deficiency in essential oils appears as hair loss, lifeless hair, dandruff or brittle hair. The above symptoms occur because EFAs are a vital component of every human cell and the body needs them to balance hormones and insulate nerve cells.

Omega 3 is found in oily fish, such as tuna, mackerel and salmon; it is also found in walnuts and dark green leafy vegetables. Omega 6 is found in nuts and seeds, especially linseed, pumpkin and sesame seed oils and also in evening primrose oil.

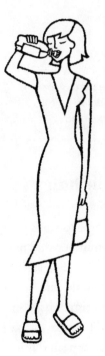

- Vitamin B foods. These are needed not only to convert the omega oils in the body but also to support protein in the hair. Vitamin B can be found in brown bread, brown rice, oats and eggs.
- Vitamin A foods. Dark green veggies and zinc (found in beans and shellfish) will both help to prevent scalp problems and are crucial for hair growth.
- Vitamin C and beta-carotene foods, such as citrus fruits and carrots. These help protect the hair and encourage hair growth.
- Vitamin E foods, such as avocados and peanut butter, will help make hair glossy and shiny.

Step two: protect your hair from the environment

UV rays from the sun attack the proteins in hair, leaving you more hairbear than hair goddess.

- In order for sun-kissed hair to look its best you need to protect it in the sun. Skin sunblocks don't work, as they need living cells to work (interesting fact if you didn't know – your hair is actually dead). For best results experts suggest using a physical block with zinc or titanium oxide, as these will reflect harmful rays. Though for maximum sunscreening wear a hat!

- To avoid dehydrated hair when you swim – usually the result of sea water and/or chlorine – coat your hair with a conditioner that repels water before you swim. Go for a product containing glycerine or petroleum, as these will coat the hair and stop the water getting in.

myth

Conditioning in the sun helps. Untrue. Slapping on conditioner on the beach or after you've been swimming locks in the salt and chlorine and helps fry, not condition hair. It's really the perfect recipe for a frenzied hairbear look.

Step three: learn to wash your hair properly

What? I hear you cry. You already know how to wash your hair – but do you? Hairdressers say the number-one mistake people make is overdoing the shampoo. For starters shampoo is a mixture of detergent, perfume and water designed to rid your hair of oil, dirt and grimy bits. Some brands come with added keratin designed to make the hair feel shiny and buoyant, others have volumisers, and thickeners. To choose, go for one that suits your hair colour, type and 'problem'.

- Massage your scalp. It not only stimulates the hair follicles, sending pleasure waves through your body and boosting circulation, but it will also help get rid of oil and skin flakes. This in turn will prevent pores from clogging and will promote hair growth. Massage before shampooing, or as you lather.

- We all need only one wash with a dollop of shampoo the size of a ten pence piece (more if your hair is extra long). Even if your scalp is oily, washing with more shampoo will encourage more oil, not less.
- Rinse thoroughly. This means really rinse not until the lather has gone but until you can hear your hair squeak.

Step four: condition right

Conditioners basically lubricate the hair shaft and are great for all types of hair, especially damaged hair.

- If your hair is excessively dry and damaged, try using a leave-in conditioner in addition to the one you use after washing.
- Deep condition, i.e. apply a hair mask once every two weeks if your hair needs extra help. Experts suggest opting for one with panthenol (vitamin B$_5$), which can penetrate the hair shaft and give you shiny hair.
- Condition once and rinse out properly (use the same technique as for washing).

Step five: dry your hair properly

How you dry your hair will affect its appearance and condition so it's worth practising care.

- Wait before you blow-dry. Ever notice how hairdressers wait until your hair is fairly dry before drying it? Well, it's not because of time issues, but because they know hair that's 80 per cent dry will end up less damaged.
- Pat dry by patting the water out of it; don't rub towel-wet hair. Vigorously rubbing your scalp will just tangle the wet hair, turning it into an unruly mess that will break when you comb it out.
- Use heat wisely. Imagine if you blitzed your hands with hot air every time you washed them. In no time they'd be chapped, sensitive and dry, so bear in mind the same happens to your scalp. Turn the hairdryer down and part blow-dry with cooler air. This will not only add volume but also protect your scalp.
- Condition before blow-drying. Hair loses about a third of its natural moisture when blown dry, but if you protect your hair first with a conditioner, heat can improve the health of your hair by forcing the moisturiser to penetrate into the hair.

DIY hair disasters

Colouring

One in three Britons colour their hair, and whether it's for beauty reasons or to cover the grey bits, we shell out millions of pounds a year on dye. But what exactly are we rubbing into our hair every six weeks? If some studies are to be believed it's not something particularly good for the scalp or our health. Reports vary, but the consensus seems to be:

read the instructions carefully and patch-test and you'll be fine using a colourant.

However to dye successfully:

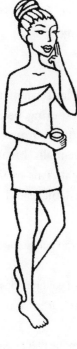

Do a 48-hour patch test: everyone should be doing this test every single time they use a hair dye; no matter if they've used that same brand 50–100 times before. This is because you can suddenly become allergic to a product.

Follow the instructions: if it says keep on for 20 minutes don't try to enhance the colour by going for 35, as this will do little but irritate your scalp. At the same time pick a suitable shade change to shift your hair colour. Don't attempt to go from blonde to black in one go. If you're unsure, speak to a hairdresser first.

Watch for a reaction: the areas of reaction to look out for are: a local reaction, which is an instant burning from the bleach, or a secondary reaction, which is a delayed one that occurs 24 hours after a tint or colour has been put on your hair. This is signified by intense itching, blistering and eventual broken skin from the itching. Other signs to watch out for are: feeling faint, swelling of the face, lips, hairline, swelling of the tongue, vomiting, diarrhoea, and any type of asthmatic symptoms. If you respond this way wash the product off immediately and seek medical advice and help.

Try a natural-based hair colourant: these are a good option if you're worried about potential chemical allergies. Salons such as Aveda use plant-based dyes, which don't contain any petrochemicals, plus Aveda colourists will always do the vital 48-hour patch test before application. However, hair colouring, like any product with a chemical basis, is never going to be completely 100 per cent safe. While severe health risks are very remote, it's also worth noting that if you want a coloured sheen to your hair, chemicals are just part of the whole package.

Chemical processes

You don't have to be a genius to know that straightening and perming is harder on the hair than colouring, because when you chemically change the hair's texture – from curly to straight or vice versa – you are essentially breaking down the hair's structure and rebuilding it. This weakens the hair, making it more prone to breaks, damage and dryness. If you're going to do it:

- Have it done professionally where an expert can gauge the health of your hair before they begin.
- If you're doing it at home, never do anything if your hair has just been coloured, as you'll be breaking down the hair twice and doubling the damage.
- Beware of redying. Lightening hair is brutal to the hair as bleach strips it of its natural melanin.

- Take your hairdresser's advice. If he advises against it, he's telling you for a good reason.

myth

Brushing your hair 100 strokes a day makes it healthy and shiny. Untrue. You don't need to be addicted to brushing to maintain healthy hair. While brushing can stimulate the scalp, two or three brushes a day is sufficient to maintain shine and suppleness.

Dandruff

tip

If you have a colour disaster – don't attempt to correct it yourself by dyeing it again, as this will weaken the hair. Always see a hair-dresser to see what your options are.

A flaking scalp – dandruff – can stem from a variety of things including stress, weather changes, and hormonal fluctuations. More often than not it's the result of stress, which changes the balance of the scalp's secretions. Persistent dandruff (dandruff that lasts for more than two weeks) is another problem altogether and is usually caused by a yeast or fungal infection. In some cases it isn't even dandruff but another skin condition, such as eczema, psoriasis or ringworm. If you're worried, see your doctor for help before you try any anti-dandruff shampoos, as he will give you a prescription for a stronger medicated shampoo. For a natural response try eating omega 3 essential fatty acids found in oily fish, which help prevent dandruff and eczema.

Body hair: keeping it, plucking it, shaving it, and zapping it

OK, this is the one type of hair you don't want to grow in abundance and keep shiny and glossy, which is why there are a variety of ways to zap it. Some techniques work better on certain areas of the body. Some work well all over, but most people go for a combined approach. Experiment and see what works best for you.

Bleaching: best for the upper lip

Good if you have relatively fair skin, but for zapping dark hairs on dark skin you could end up with a blonde moustache. Bleaching needs to be done only once every month (sometimes longer) but can be messy and time-consuming.

Depilatory creams: best for the body

These are cheap and easy to use but must always be patch-tested for 24 hours before use, just in case the cream is too strong for your skin. This method is long-lasting and stubble-free, but it's messy and time-consuming, so not good for girls on the run.

Laser hair removal and electrolysis: best for facial hair and the bikini line

Removing hair using a laser is a relatively new cosmetic procedure that can end up costing you the earth, as you usually need ten sessions for it to work. The hair is zapped at the root by a laser, which then slows down hair growth. Some companies promise that this is permanent but this isn't the case, as even though a hair follicle is destroyed, nothing can stop a new hair from growing back in its place. The results do vary from person to person, and in some cases are fairly useless. Electrolysis works on a similar principle: an electrical current is applied to the hair root. Again this is expensive and time-consuming, and the hair will still grow back.

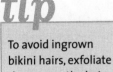

tip

To avoid ingrown bikini hairs, exfoliate the area as the hair starts to regrow. This will stop the follicles curling in on themselves.

Plucking: best for eyebrows

If you want neat eyebrows then follow the line of the brow and gently pluck the hairs underneath the brow. Plucking between the brows gets rid of that mono-eyebrow look, but don't overdo it or else you'll resemble a rather startled bird.

Sugaring: best for legs

An age-old Eastern technique that is very like waxing, sugaring also has a similar pain value and regrowth effect.

How to pluck your brows

- Invest in a good pair of tweezers as they will not only grasp the hair more accurately but also will be handy when trying to get hold of those fine hairs.
- Do follow fashion: brows change with hairstyles and clothes. Think of the thin pencil line of the 60s compared to the fuller brow we have now.
- If you overpluck, allow the hair to grow back before reshaping again. It will be unruly for a while but worth it.
- Don't pluck from above. Always remove hair from below, as this is how to get an arch.

Shaving: best for lower legs and underarms

When all else fails the best friend to a lazy girl is her razor. It's fast, it's efficient and if you do it right it can last for more than a few days.

First a few shaving no-nos:

- Never share your razor. A good way to catch an infection or spread one is to use the same blade as someone else. Buy your own.
- Never shave your face unless you want to end up with a five o'clock shadow (and you will).
- Don't use a razor on dry skin unless you want to go for a hacked-up look.

- Be careful where you shave. Legs and underarms are fine, but thighs and bikini line can lead to a nasty scratchy feeling as the hair grows back (not sexy).
- Change your razor blades regularly, as they become blunt fairly fast.
- Moisturise after shaving, it will not only soothe the legs but also improve their look.

myth

Shaving makes your hair grow back stronger. Untrue. An old wives' tale; it may feel as if the hair is now stronger and there's more of it, but all you're feeling are the sharp edges of the hair as it comes through – the result of the way you have shaved and nothing else.

Waxing: best for bikini line, legs, eyebrows and upper lip

Salon waxing is the current celebrity favourite and is better than home kits for a variety of reasons. Firstly, it's more thorough, especially around your bikini line, and secondly, a beautician can do it more efficiently and therefore decrease the pain factor.

Pros to waxing are softer hair growth, longer-lasting hair-free days, and less of a hassle on a day-to-day basis.

Avoiding the ouch! factor

- Don't use a sunbed or sunbathe before going for a wax. When your skin is hot, the wax heats up, which can lead to potential scars and more pain when the strip is peeled off.
- Avoid waxing when you are premenstrual, as you are more sensitive to pain just before your period begins.
- Avoid working out before a wax. Again, this heats up the skin.
- Relax before they let rip, tensing up in anticipation of pain puts your muscles on red alert and worsens the effect.
- Don't let things overgrow. If you want to go down the waxing path, go regularly. Letting your hair overgrow means longer sessions and more pain, and post-wax soreness.
- Exfoliate between waxes (especially on your bikini line) – it stops ingrown hairs.
- If you do get ingrown hairs (hair that loops back under the skin instead of poking out of the follicle) they'll usually appear as nasty red bumps that have to be tweezed gently or released with a bikini-zone product that has salicylic acid within it.
- Moisturise after waxing to soothe the area – try aloe vera.

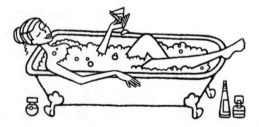

20 ways to keep your extremities looking good

Greying around the temples is a sign that you're deficient in these foods.

1 Load up on vitamins
Not only great for your immune system but will also boost hair growth, nail growth and skin repair.

2 Sunbathe with hair sunscreen, not conditioner, on your hair
Conditioners are for use with damp not dry heat. The heat of the sun will therefore fry your hair, due to the oils in the conditioner.

3 Take painkillers before a wax
Swallow two 40 minutes before you go and your wax will be relatively pain-free.

4 Avoid premature greying
By eating more vitamin B foods.

5 Go barefoot
This will help exercise the 26 bones and 20 muscles that make up your foot. Concentrate on walking heel to toe.

6 Do something about your emotional stress
This not only aids hair loss and spots but also is a common cause of smelly feet (as the sweat glands on the soles of the feet respond to emotion the fastest).

7 Don't have a leg wax the day before your holiday
Have your pre-beach wax earlier, as skin can take at least 48 hours to settle down, and if you suddenly expose it to the sun, you're asking for bumpy skin.

8 Never swim after a bikini wax
Ideally wait three days before swimming in chlorinated water or your newly bare bikini line will become irritated, red and lumpy.

9 Protect coloured hair in the sun
Heard the one about a girl's hair turning green in the pool? Well it's true. If you have coloured hair use a sunscreen that's waterproof and a shampoo that has a UV filter to protect coloured hair.

10 Rub as you wash
Always give your head a massage when washing it. It increases the blood supply to the head and visibly makes hair more bouncy. Use cold water for the last rinse; it makes hair shinier.

11 Get to grips with those tricky hairs
If you are plucking (let's not say where!) and you come across a really stubborn hair, put some concealer on the end of the tweezers; it really helps to get a grip and you'll yank it out with no trouble.

12 Moisturise dry hair with a banana or avocado mask
Mash ripe banana with a teaspoon of almond oil and then massage into dry or damp hair. Rinse off after 20 minutes for perfect, glossy hair.

13 Scrub your feet
Make up your own body scrub with 45 ml (3 tablespoons) of sea salt and 250 ml (1 cup) of almond oil. Mix with water to make a paste and then massage on to your feet and rinse. Then rub aloe vera cream into your feet for perfect toes.

14 Soothe cracked heels
Limit time spent in mules and flip-flops as the slapping action aids cracking. For super-smooth feet, go for a foot wrap. Massage the above scrub into your feet and then wrap in cling film and pull some socks on. Watch TV for two hours and then rinse off.

15 Get some more sleep
This is the cheapest and most relaxing of beauty treatments. Studies now show that eight hours of sleep a night not only helps your hair, nail and skin cells regenerate but also helps to

relax your muscles so you awake looking and feeling years younger.

16 Avoid limp sun hair
Your hair goes floppy because your scalp is perspiring and mixing with your hair's natural oils. The trick is to put some toner on to a cotton-wool pad and rub it along your parting and forehead to dry up excess oil.

17 Make a pedicure last longer
Apply a thin layer of oil to not-quite-dry polish. Then reapply a thin layer of topcoat once a week.

18 Wipe astringent surgical spirit between your toes
It mops up sweat, helps you avoid athlete's foot and keeps your toes nice and dry.

19 Beware of tiny fibres
Use 100 per cent cotton balls or else you'll be left with fibre fuzz under your nail varnish.

20 Get your eyebrows shaped by a professional
It will give you an instant facelift, as a shaped brow defines your eyes, and gives you a wider, clearer look.

chapter 3

Keep young and beautiful

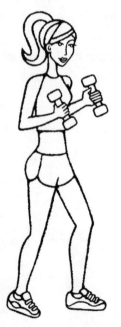

Beauty products and make-up are essential tools for the lazy girl, simply because they allow the slobbiest and the most unhealthiest of girls to appear as if they are glowing with health and beauty. Bad skin and bags under your eyes? Just slap on some foundation and, bingo! You're ten years younger. Greasy, lank hair? Tie it up, stick a flower in and immediately you have supermodel locks. Nasty nails? Stick on real-looking falsies and no one will ever know. Thankfully, for most of us the list of cover-ups is endless, and as long as you have the money you can look beautiful and gorgeous well into your thirties and forties.

The only problem is (and you knew one was coming, didn't you?) that if you rely solely on products to make you beautiful, sooner or later you're going to be in BIG trouble!

Time puts its mark on everyone, and if you're a party girl who gives no thought to the future or her insides, the mark's going to be bigger than you think. Luckily there's a lazy way round the ageing problem: (1) Accept that no matter what you do you're going to get older, and (2) Note that with a bit of extra effort you can actually age gracefully; as in look beautiful when you're old, rather than be beautiful until you get old.

Short-term beauty — how to knock ten years off your age

Get your hair cut: long hair ages you faster than short. So get some layers cut into your hair for a more flattering and younger look. Blow-dry hair away from the face or tie it back for maximum youthful effect.

Go for a natural facelift: by having your eyebrows plucked and shaped. It will lift the eye and give your face a fresh appearance.

Buy a new foundation: swap powder for cream and you'll not only have a smoother finish but also have younger-looking skin.

Wear a glossier lipstick: it will plump out thinning lips.

Stand up straight: you'll really look as if you have lost 10 pounds. This means shoulders back, stomach in and head up.

Buy a good body moisturiser: one that offers the best in shimmer and moisture to both make your skin glow with radiance and feel good.

Drink eight glasses of water a day: it will give you the energy of an 18-year-old.

Long-lasting beauty equals diet and exercise

The real trick to long-lasting beauty is simply to look after your health. Yawn you may, but let your insides go to pot and no matter how gorgeous and sexy you look now, gravity will eventually pull you downwards. If you've adopted a sedentary lifestyle (69 per cent of men and 54 per cent of women don't exert themselves on a regular basis) it will also happen faster than you think. In truth, the implications of being a human sofa are staggering so if you do one thing for the sake of your beauty make it exercise, as it's this which keeps your heart healthy, counteracts the pull of gravity and boosts your immune system; all fantastic beauty boosters.

Work out just three times a week and it will not only decrease the age of your body but it will also boost your sex drive and delay the body's natural degeneration, i.e. you'll look, feel and be younger than you actually are. Better still, it will give you some extra benefits, such as a better body, healthier skin and maybe even the much-desired flat stomach (a good excuse to finally bin your big knickers).

Beauty-boosting exercise tips

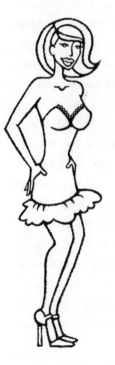

- Do 20–40 minutes of vigorous aerobic exercise three times a week. Aim to make sure your heart rate is working at the right intensity (a good indication is being breathless). Too breathless to talk? You're in the right zone.
- Do some weight-bearing exercise. This is essential for women because female bone mass peaks at the age of 35 and then declines by 1 per cent a year. If you don't exercise you could be one of the one in three women who end up with the brittle-bone disease, osteoporosis, which beauty-wise will mean stooped posture, loss of height and bones that literally crumble when you fall. Just 15 minutes of weight-bearing exercise (walking, running, free weights) a day will keep you strong for life.
- Stabilise your core. If you are neglecting to strengthen your core muscle groups (the ones that run around the body, like a corset) you're more likely to end up bent over with pain as you get older. Fifteen minutes a day will keep you straight and lean, plus avoiding backache and perpetual tiredness.
- Stop doing the sit-up. If you've been doing the traditional sit-up and getting nowhere fast it's time to face that it doesn't work simply because it engages the wrong tummy muscles. Luckily, an American exercise scientist, from San Diego State University, tested the 13 most popular abdominal exercises for effectiveness and came up with the top four belly-busters. To get the

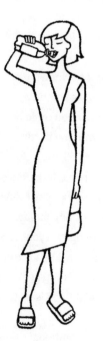

desired effects do three sets of all four exercises every day for 15 minutes.

- **The bicycle:** the aim here is to pretend you're riding an imaginary cycle while lying on the floor. To get it right, press your lower back into the floor and put your hands behind your head. Bring your knees up to a 45-degree angle and slowly move your legs in a bicycle motion, while touching your left elbow to your right knee, and your right elbow to your left knee.

- **Knee raises:** sit on the edge of a stable chair, knees bent and feet flat on the floor; hold on to the sides of the chair. Tighten your tummy, lean back slightly and lift your feet several centimetres off the floor. Now in a steady movement pull knees in towards your chest and crunch your upper body forward. Lower your feet to the original position and repeat.

- **Army sit-up:** lie down, knees bent, feet together and anchored under a steady couch. Loop a towel around the back of your neck and hold each end. Contract your tummy and lift your shoulders and then your back curling all the way up and then lower almost to the floor and repeat. If it's too hard, just lift your upper body off the floor and build up to the above.

- **Ball lift:** lie back, holding a tennis ball in your hands, and raise your arms towards the ceiling, with your legs extended together and feet flexed. Tighten your tummy muscles and bottom, and lift your shoulders and head a few centimetres off the ground. Make sure the ball goes towards the ceiling and not forwards.

- Aim to sweat. The aim with all aerobic exercise is to sweat. If you're not sweating you're not working hard enough. The better shape you're in the more you sweat and the sooner you start sweating when you exercise. It may leave you looking as red as a tomato but it's good for you, so go for it.

Beauty-boosting diet tips

Survive on takeaways, yo-yo diet and sit on your sofa eating chocolate every night and you don't need an expert to tell you you're going to age quickly and badly. The implications of eating badly are staggering for both your looks and the ageing process. Think muscle loss, weak bones, lethargy, wrinkles, a sagging face and age-related diseases, such as atherosclerosis (hardening of the arteries). By comparison, eating a diet rich in protein, complex carbohydrates, fruit and vegetables, as well as some of your favourites, will help your body stay in youthful shape.

- Eat plenty of green leafy vegetables, such as broccoli, cabbage and spinach, and dark fruit, such as plums and berries, as they are full of antioxidants, which fight the ageing process and help you to look and feel young.
- Choose lean meats, salads, vegetables, chicken and fish. Oily fish is particularly good as it's full of essential fatty acids (omega 3 and 6), which protect your heart and your skin and keep age-related illnesses away.

- Choose soya products as they contain isoflavones, which boost hormone levels and protect against cancer and osteoporosis.
- Foods packed with vitamins A, C and E are essential as they help maintain the structure of the skin. Try apricots, watercress, eggs, tomatoes, almonds, avocados and oatmeal.
- Take an age-defying supplement. Ginkgo biloba is an excellent brain booster, selenium reduces the risk of heart disease, and coenzyme Q10 is essential for healthy skin.

tip

Working out helps you stay young, but don't over do it. Exercising everyday at a high intensity will age your looks and will leave you tired, exhausted and prone to illness.

- Eat some protein every day. About 25 per cent of your daily food intake should come from protein because it's essential for building bones, healthy teeth, hair and nails. It's also vital for healthy blood and maintaining your blood sugar levels. The best sources are chicken, fish, soya products, milk and eggs.
- Eat carbohydrates every day. There are two types of carbohydrates: complex and simple. A simple carbohydrate is any grain that has been processed to remove it from its original state; for example, bread or pasta. Eat too much of the simple carbohydrates and you'll feel tired and sluggish because this kind of food is converted into sugar very quickly by the body.
- Eat fat every day. Not all fat is bad for your health. The body needs unsaturated fat for cell growth, fertility, healthy periods and skin. It's also essential for hormones and healthy bones. This means you can't afford to cut all fat from your diet. The essential fats to take are omega 3 and 6 fatty acids found in oily fish, nuts and seeds. Deficiency signs are dry skin and mood swings.

myth

You can never be too thin. Untrue. You can when it comes to beauty and ageing. Apart from the fact that your skin will start to hang if you get too thin, being too skinny depletes oestrogen, the hormone needed to keep you looking young and healthy. Oestrogen needs body fat to do its work; diet too far and your body fat will drop out of sight leaving you looking and feeling like a has-been.

How to look beautiful forever

Buy an anti-ageing cream

You honestly get what you pay for when it comes to anti-ageing creams. Not that I am advocating spending your life savings on a pot the size of your thumbnail. If you look after your skin, eat well, use sunscreen and don't succumb to too many bad habits, you'll never have to buy one. However, for those who want a bit of extra help or some repair work, here's the low-down on anti-agers.

Anti-ageing creams do work, but not to the extent most people wish they would, i.e. they won't make you look 20 years old if you're 35! Ingredients contained within the creams such as alpha hydroxy acids (AHAs), antioxidants, vitamins and yeast extracts make your skin appear younger by working on the skin's surface. Most form a protective barrier and so eventually reveal a brighter complexion.

Anti-ageing ingredients

Antioxidants, also known as vitamins A, C and E: most of the creams on the market now contain these vitamins. Though it's worth noting they do not sink into the lower layers of your skin but remain on the outside protecting against environmental hazards. So it's best to get your antioxidants through your diet.

Kinetin: the ideal ingredient for sensitive skin, as it is said to leave skin feeling healthy and refreshed.

Grapeseed extract: this supposedly helps fight against environmental damage by acting as a barrier.

Glucosamine: young skin has a cell turnover of 28 days, but in older skin this can slow to 40 days making skin look dry and dull. Glucosamine works as an exfoliator within a cream to help these new cells come through.

Soya: ideal for firming-up skin, especially good for dry skin. Again, best taken in your diet rather than via a cream.

Marine collagen: also known as seaweed and elastin, it is said to be excellent for nourishing the skin.

Arnica: soothing and stimulating for sensitive skin.

Anti-ageing make-up tips

Make-up can make you look ten years younger or ten years older, and the line between the two is fine. To help yourself:

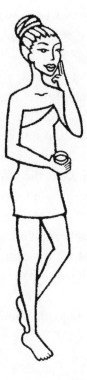

- Avoid thick make-up bases. You may want to use your foundation as Polyfilla but it won't work. If anything you'll accentuate lines and wrinkles. Instead, apply your foundation in thin layers and preferably with a make-up sponge to get an even look.
- Don't make up your eyes to resemble those of a panda. Heavy eyeliner and dark shadow can make wrinkled lids look saggy not sexy.
- Do wear gloss to make your lips look fuller (just a dot in the centre of the lips will do the trick, don't go for plastic Barbie lips).
- Do blot your face with a tissue after applying powder so it doesn't just lie on your face (and avoid putting powder under your eyes where it can accentuate fine lines).
- Don't overlash your eyelashes – you'll resemble a startled spider.
- Good summer camouflage for days when you don't want to wear full make-up but still need to cover up: rub some foundation with some SPF moisturiser into your skin. It will give you a more radiant and even look.

Make the most of your hormones

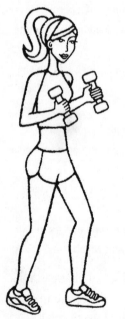

Hands up if you've seen those adverts promising miracle creams that will whittle away your wrinkles and leave you looking 18 years old forever. Well, I'm sure you don't need me to tell you what a load of old nonsense that is (see above for what they can do). If you want to restore ageing skin to its former glory the only thing that will work is a facelift and you're not going to find that in a bottle, no matter how expensive.

But before you give up on ever doing anything to your skin again, bear in mind your skin will stay firm and elastic until you reach your mid-thirties, if you do everything mentioned so far: i.e. keep out of the sun and stay clear of cigarettes, take exercise and maintain a healthy diet. After this point, being female will eventually affect the way you look because of the female hormone, oestrogen (although other hormones also get involved, see below).

A good supply of oestrogen means soft, supple, healthy and resilient skin. A low supply means the opposite, and unfortunately, levels naturally start to decrease at the onset of menopause.

To keep skin soft and supple throughout your life, increase oestrogen by:

Eating phyto-oestrogens: these are natural plant-based oestrogens found in citrus fruits, wheat, oats and rhubarb, and green and yellow vegetables. It's well documented that Japanese women, who eat a diet rich in plant oestrogens, have fewer problems at menopause when their oestrogen levels fall.

Eating isoflavones: these are known to decrease the risk of hormone-related cancers and reduce menopausal symptoms, all caused by falling oestrogen levels. Found in soya bean products, such as tofu.

Taking phyto-nutrient herbs: these are herbs that balance hormones. Liquorice boosts oestrogen when levels are too low and inhibits levels when they are too high. Ginseng also helps by balancing the body's adrenal (stress) hormones, which in turn affect the production of oestrogen.

tip

Less is more when you start getting older. Less obvious make up and less fussy hair styles!

Human growth hormone (HGH)

This hormone is produced in the pituitary gland and stimulates the growth of bone and muscle in the body. Unfortunately, like a variety of hormones, it declines after the age of 31. From here on in it falls by 24 per cent per decade, and by 60 years it's cut by 75 per cent. Bad news for us because the many physical and mental changes associated with ageing such as saggy skin, an increase in weight and lack of energy are directly linked to declining levels.

Growth hormone replacement is said to restore hair

growth, reduce wrinkles, boost fat metabolism and kick-start your sex drive.

How to increase HGH in your body

Exercise: strenuous activity for 30 minutes every day will boost levels in the body. Exercising when hungry has been shown to raise HGH faster.

Diet: eat a healthy diet, with a mix of protein, vegetables, fruit and complex carbohydrate such as potatoes, rice and pasta. Limit levels of processed foods.

Amino acid L-arginine: this naturally helps to increase the production of HGH. It's found in protein foods, such as oily fish, cottage cheese, bananas, soya and lean meat.

Dehydroepiandrosterone (DHEA)

Produced by the adrenal glands, DHEA is the mother of all chemicals, as it can transform into almost any other hormone in the body, including the two essential sex hormones: testosterone and oestrogen. DHEA is particularly important to our sex lives because it influences who we find attractive, as well as increasing libido, preserving lean body mass and producing the pheromones which emit our sexual scent to others. The bad news is levels decline massively from the age of 30, which is one of the reasons why DHEA has emerged as a leading anti-ageing supplement in Europe. However, as yet it's not available in the UK or USA because there is a concern that there is a link between supplements and liver problems.

How to increase DHEA in your body

Vigorous exercise: this can boost DHEA, but, for a good response, you need to do at least 30 minutes of fast-paced exercise a day for approximately one month.

Meditation: this also elevates DHEA by lowering stress levels, as shown by studies at the Maharishi University – a centre for transcendental meditation.

Wild yam supplement: this contains a natural steroid called diosgenin, which converts to DHEA. However, research is limited so the only way to judge its efficiency is to take it for six weeks and see if it works.

Lowering your alcohol levels: this will also boost DHEA. Studies show that alcohol injections reduce brain levels of DHEA within 30 minutes. Recovery to normal levels then takes four hours.

De-stress your looks

There's good stress and there's bad stress. Good stress is the stuff that gets you fired up for an interview, makes you

myth

Good genes will keep you young-looking. Untrue. The look of your skin is 30 per cent genetics and 70 per cent environment. So while good genes can help you look younger for longer, they won't halt the ageing process.

excited about new prospects and leaves a happy smile on your face. Bad stress, on the other hand, gives you that deep groove in your forehead, gritted teeth at night and the feeling that no amount of sleep will ever leave you feeling refreshed. Whether you're adept at spotting your bad stress signs or not, your looks can give you the red-alert signals to watch for:

- Skin conditions such as rosacea (see Chapter 1), eczema, and psoriasis (see Chapter 2) are all stress-related.
- Hives (urticaria), skin rashes and sweat rashes are caused by overproductive sweat glands spurred on by stress levels.
- More dandruff, caused by increased inflammation from the hair follicles, is a by-product of tension and worry.
- Greasy hair and acne. Stress increases the activity of your sebaceous glands.
- Grey hair. Though there is little scientific evidence to back this up, some experts believe that when you're stressed, the body uses up quantities of vitamin B in the body. And as there is a

connection between vitamin B depletion and greying hair you're likely to see a change of hair colour.

- Hair loss. What usually happens is you go through a stressful event, which at the time makes your hair stop growing, and then about eight weeks later you notice a greater hair loss than usual. The hair will start growing again naturally, but if you're worried see your doctor to rule out other conditions, such as an iron deficiency.

To de-stress your life for the sake of your looks, firstly don't work too hard. The perfect advice for the lazy girl, but too many hours sitting at a computer, not only kills your posture and your brain cells but also ages you faster.

Secondly do something relaxing, such as swimming, yoga or lying in the sunshine. Just ten minutes a day will help you sleep better, rejuvenate your skin and help you to breathe better, which in turn will send more oxygen round to your vital organs. Thirdly, RELAX about your life. Easier said than done, but your facial muscles will stay on red alert if you don't learn to relax. So unless you want grooves

tip

Youthfulness is all in your attitude. No matter what your age, be optimistic about life and the years will drop off you.

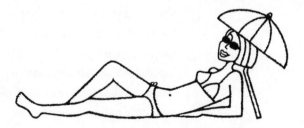

in your forehead, frown lines across your mouth and pursed lips forever, here are some fast ways to relax:

Instant beauty stress relief

- Breathe diaphragmatically. Inhale through your nose and push your diaphragm out as you breathe in, then hold your breath and slowly exhale for the same time. Do this ten times (build up to it or else you'll feel too relaxed) and repeat every day for a month. You'll be amazed at the transformation in your face and energy levels.

- Massage your face. It sounds weird but have you ever noticed how children rub their faces when they're tired? They know the secret to waking up is to get some circulation going and to wake up those fixed facial muscles. If you ever wonder why your face feels so odd after work, take a look in the mirror as you work to see your 'concentration look'. If it's like most people's it's likely to be head jutted forward, jaw fixed, tongue on roof of mouth, and mouth downturned.

- Take a walk – preferably outside your office. It's good for your mind and your looks, as office air is nasty stuff as far as your complexion is concerned. Experts suggest getting up and stretching at least once an hour, with a ten-minute break at least once every three hours.

- Pamper yourself. Why wait for the day when you're ten pounds lighter, have a boyfriend, more money, more time etc. Do it now. Go on, you deserve it. Instead of spending your money on nothing in particular, pay for an aromatherapy massage, a reflexology treatment or a home spa kit (see Chapter 7). It will leave you looking a million dollars.

- Take a power nap. Feeling exhausted? Too tired to think? Does your head feel too heavy for your shoulders (which are probably up around your ears)? Are your eyes puffy and your skin pallid? If so, you need a ten-minute power nap. Studies show ten minutes is all you need to rejuvenate yourself (any more and you go into too deep a sleep). So set your computer alarm and nod off.

- Treat yourself to some good bath products. Soaking yourself in a bath filled with expensive oils and foam works as a relaxant on two fronts: one, hot water helps soothe tense muscles (soak for at least ten minutes), and two, indulging yourself helps reduce mental stress.

- Jump on the sofa. Yes, couch-potato time is also invaluable de-stress time. Lying back and thinking of nothing (or watching bad TV) not only helps your body to relax but also eases facial muscles (giving you a mini-facelift) and helps you cut off from worry and tension.

Get your beauty sleep

The cheapest and most rewarding beauty treatment you'll ever find is a good night's sleep. That's sleep that lasts for eight hours, is not interrupted and is not fuelled by alcohol. Yup, it's not called beauty sleep for nothing. Part of the benefit of sleep comes from the fact that after a hard day's work your body needs to recuperate and literally rest.

Throughout the night our bodies follow a sleep pattern.

tip

They call it beauty sleep for a reason. Get less than 7 hours a night and you're asking for dull skin, bags under your eyes and lank hair.

The first 90–100 minutes are non-REM sleep – essential to boost our energy levels after being awake for 16–17 hours. REM (rapid eye movement) sleep, which happens later in the night, is a stage of vigorous brain activity; this plays a major role in boosting our performance and sexual and learning functions. Do yourself out of either and you're asking for beauty trouble, as the release of growth hormones in your body will slow down. These are the hormones that step up cell renewal (essential for good skin), boost energy stores (essential for circulation and getting rid of dark circles around your eyes) and help generate hair and nail growth. Get too little sleep and you'll be left with tired skin, bags under your eyes, low energy and loss of concentration.

Boost your beauty sleep

- Make your bedroom sleep-friendly. Don't watch TV in bed; this revs up adrenalin levels, making it hard for you to sleep or making you think you can't sleep without watching TV.
- Make your bed sleep-friendly. Get rid of too many cushions, throws and blankets. Being too hot will hinder your sleep and too many pillows are bad for your sleeping posture.
- Keep a window open for fresh air. This is good for your breathing.

- Think about your problems an hour before you go to bed and then relax in a hot bath so your mind is not racing as you try to sleep.
- If you can't sleep, get up after 20 minutes and do something until you feel tired.
- Don't eat foods that are hard to digest (dairy, fatty foods, spicy foods) after 8 p.m.
- Try putting some valerian or lavender essential oil on to your pillow.
- Don't oversleep – it's as bad as lack of sleep, as it knocks your body clock off, and means you wake up feeling lethargic and looking puffy in the face.
- Beware of too much caffeine; it is found in coffee, colas, some chocolate bars, tea and in some painkillers.
- Buy some earplugs to shut out a partner's snoring and incidental noise from the street. At the same time make sure your room is dark enough.
- Avoid aerobic exercise after 7 p.m., as it revs the body up, instead of calming it down for sleep.

20 ways
to stay young and
beautiful

1 Improve your posture
Most of us spend eight hours a day in a slumped, slouched position – little wonder then that our bellies flop forward and our shoulders hunch when we stand up. So if you do nothing else to help yourself look young, make sure you improve your posture.

2 Think sexy
During sexual fantasies small releases of HGH (human growth hormone) are released. This helps reduce fatty tissue and helps the body to stay younger-looking.

3 Wear a lighter shade of lipstick
Dark colours make the lips look thinner. Apply a dab of gloss to the centre of your lower lip to make the lips look plumper and fuller.

4 Laugh more
A University of Southern California study found that laughing boosts your immune system by 25 per cent and at the same time slows down the ageing process.

5 Eat more fruit
According to research published in the British Medical Journal (BMJ), consuming fresh fruit daily has the greatest effect on longevity, thanks to its cancer-fighting properties.

6 Surround yourself with friends
Being sociable and creating your own personal 'family' will, says a study in the BMJ, help you live longer and more happily than loners.

7 Stop worrying
Stress studies show anxiety speeds up the ageing process.

8 Have regular sex
It will help you feel and look young, thanks to the release of hormones sex

generates, by reducing your risk of premature death by 36 per cent.

9 Drink some milk

It sounds dull, but calcium is needed as you get older to maintain the look of hair, teeth and nails. If you hate milk, go for spinach and broccoli.

10 Take ten minutes for yourself twice a day

Watch TV, close your eyes, listen to music, do some yoga or simply do nothing. You'll be amazed at how refreshed it leaves you looking.

11 Keep your concealer light around the eyes

Too dark and you'll give your eyes a crinkled look. Too heavy and you'll look like you're wearing a mask. Go for a light shade that blends as you rub it in.

12 Buy body moisturisers that also have anti-ageing qualities

Don't forget all the other crêpey bits, such as your neck, elbows and knees. Buy a cream that will enhance your skin, leaving it feeling firmer to the touch.

13 Do some weight training

It won't leave you looking like a bodybuilder but it will give you a younger-looking body with good muscle definition. The big bonus being the more muscle you have the more calories you burn.

14 Avoid a scraggy neck

Imagine a string attached to the top of your head pulling you upwards (not outwards, thin chin should be tucked in) so that the neck muscles have to work to support the head, keeping them nice and firm.

15 Ditch powder-based make-up

Swap them for cream- and gloss-based make-ups, as skin with a slight sheen looks younger and healthier.

16 Eat a superfood

Broccoli, rich in antioxidants, could add five years to your life.
Oats lower cholesterol and will keep you feeling fighting fit.

Oily fish has protective benefits for your heart, your mood and your skin.

Garlic lowers blood pressure and boosts immunity.

Avocado is a good source of glutathione – an anti-ageing chemical.

17 Get up early

It's not as hard as you think. You'll be amazed at how young it makes you look and how energised it leaves you feeling all day. Studies show 5 a.m. is when energy levels are at their most powerful (though this does last until at least 7.30 a.m.).

18 Don't let your hair age you

After a certain time a hairstyle you had when you were 19 years old won't still make you look young and sexy. Don't let your hair scream 'clinging to youth'.

19 Cry more

Emotional tears contain stress hormones says The Dry Eye and Tear Research Centre in Minnesota. Alleviate your stress by crying and you'll halve your risk of stress-related disorders.

20 Go to the dentist every six months

Good tooth care can reduce your biological age by six years. This is because gum disease can also cause your arteries to swell, leading to heart disease. Plus a clean, white smile makes you look instantly younger.

chapter 4

The body beautiful aka how to look like Barbie

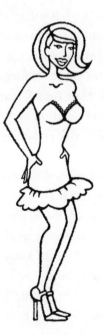

If you're a lazy girl at heart, the chances are that you've often weighed up the option of days at the gym against cosmetic surgery. After all, why try when you can have someone literally nip, tuck and pull your body into shape? This is not to say cosmetic surgery is a *must* in the lazy beauty stakes – because it's not. Many women would rather chew their toenails than pay someone to make them look like Barbie. Each to their own, but whatever your preference, cosmetic procedures are currently at the hot end of the beauty business and sell themselves on the idea that anyone can achieve beauty and perfection (at the right price of course).

Just think of the girls having bottom implants in Brazil, the women succumbing to fat-zapping and sucking in America and boob-enlarging and decreasing in the UK and you'll get the idea of how successful and everyday cosmetic surgery has become. Have enough money and you, too, can get make-up tattooed permanently on to your face. Do it enough times and you'll have the complexion of a 16-year-old for life (mind you, the rest of your body will give you away). Fed up with looking like a potato? A nip, tuck and major stomach vacuum, and bingo! You'll be thin (well, thinner)!

Jokes aside, if you're tempted, or even toying with the idea, it pays not only to be pragmatic about the amount of work you want done (if in doubt think of Michael Jackson) but also to be realistic about how surgery can transform your life. While wrinkle-free foreheads, thin thighs and bosoms that reach for the sky are only an operation away, having surgery won't make you beautiful if you genuinely feel you've been hit with the ugly stick.

What's more, surgery is addictive. Think you'll have Botox only once? Think again. Imagine you'll be happy with smaller breasts? Well, not if it draws attention to your tummy. This is why it pays to remember that beauty treatments are about making yourself feel beautiful, not about trying to appear beautiful when you feel ugly inside.

If surgery is what you want, then by all means go for it, but do it sensibly. Take some tips and ensure you don't end up with rubber-tyre lips, boobs you can rest your drinks on and a blank vacant expression.

Cosmetic surgery is not for you, if ...

- You're expecting it to change your life/find you a boyfriend and make you famous.
- You have unrealistic expectations about how it will make you look.
- You're doing it because you're too lazy to diet and take some exercise.
- If you don't intend to change your lifestyle habits afterwards (particularly important for liposuction and facial treatments).
- You have self-esteem issues.
- You think it will keep you looking and feeling young.
- You can't handle the fact you're going to get old.
- Your boyfriend wants you to have it.

Put yourself in safe hands

Whatever treatment you are going for, it pays to put yourself in safe hands and not just go for the cheapest price option, especially as the cosmetic surgery industry is still unregulated in most countries. Questions to ask pre-surgery are:

What are the risks?

The risks with cosmetic surgery are the same as the risks for any surgical procedure that you have under general anaesthetic. However, the real problem is anyone can put up a nameplate and call him or herself a cosmetic consultant. This means there is a cowboy market out there with doctors who don't have any qualifications performing procedures like Botox and liposuction. To find the best doctor, go through reputable clinics and check your doctor out with your country's official cosmetic-surgery body.

How can you find the best price?

Shop around so you can see what's available. This means looking for a reputable surgeon you feel comfortable with, so you can make an informed choice not a monetary one. If you're being offered something that sounds too good or too cheap to be true, then it probably is.

What should happen before you decide to have a procedure?

During an initial consultation a surgeon should always enquire about your general health and well-being. Plus he or she will ask about your past medical history and any medication you are taking (including alternative medication). This is to ensure you are fit and healthy for surgery. If he doesn't ask, run away ... and fast.

What if it goes wrong?

If your surgery goes wrong, your first port of call is to go back to your original surgeon for help. If you have no luck there (which is rare), see your own doctor for help.

How long will it take to recover from surgery?

Unlike treatments such as Botox and collagen implants, cosmetic surgery is not something you can nip out for at lunchtime. This means recovery is a long process. With a nose job, regular life can be resumed within a fortnight; the same is so for liposuction though bruising and swelling can take up to three months to disappear. With breast operations and tummy tucks recovery can sometimes take four to six weeks – and even longer if you want to go back to strenuous activity, such as the gym.

What are the long-term problems with surgery?

There should be no long-term problems; the only irritation factor with certain procedures is that they don't last. Botox needs to be done every three to four months, as do

tip

If a doctor doesn't check out – avoid at all costs. And if the price is too good to be true – then it's too good to be true!

collagen lip implants. Breast implants last ten years, and liposuction has a weird side effect of fat coming back in places around the site you've had sucked (especially if you load up on a fatty diet and avoid exercise).

myth

You can have surgery on the same area as many times as you like. Untrue. Not recommended by the experts. Because plastic surgery is a private procedure, even though no one can stop you from having more and more operations be aware of seeing cosmetic surgery as a miracle. It has its limitations and cannot be relied upon to transform your life. Plus the more times you work on an area the more it's likely to have scarring.

Give me that Barbie look

(Everything you'll ever need to know about cosmetic surgery)

With so many procedures available you really need to know the pros and cons of each before you can make that big decision.

Liposuction

What is it? Liposuction, the human equivalent of vacuuming, wasn't actually devised as a method to avoid dieting

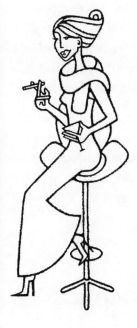

but as a way to lift off stubborn pockets of fat that wouldn't shift with exercise and diet alone. It's currently the most popular cosmetic procedure worldwide, with women having fat removed from their thighs, abdomen, hips and upper back.

Potential limitations: liposuction can eliminate as much as 3 litres (5¼ pints) of fat deposits in a given area in one go. However, the bad news is this procedure doesn't equal permanent fat removal and is not a weight-loss treatment. Not only is it more effective for people of average weight but also the fat can, and will, come back, though not in the exact spot, as fat cells are thought not to regenerate. This means if you overeat and don't exercise you'll end up with a lumpy effect around the treated area.

Which is why liposuction is not a miracle cure that will give you the body of a supermodel. Apart from the fact those gals are genetically predisposed to having lean, long bodies, there are limits, based on your size, to how many areas of the body can be operated on and how much fat can be removed.

What to expect: the operation itself has improved of late with regulations now in place to stop mass fat removal (the cause of death of a number of women in the USA). The current technique involves a hollow tubular instrument called a cannula, which is attached to a suction machine that is inserted into your body to evacuate fat. The cannula has a highly polished surface to allow it to slip between the fatty tissues with minimum effort. However, bruising, soreness and bleeding will all occur after the operation.

Liposuction works better if: you're of average weight; your skin is toned already, as liposuction can actually make flabby skin look worse; you control your weight and take up exercise after you've recovered from your operation.

Recovery time: the risks from liposuction are now very small and you can be back at work within two weeks. Swelling reduces in two days, but the new shape can take about three to six weeks to come through. Scarring is also minimal, as the incisions tend to be small slit shapes that are less than 1 cm (½ inch) long.

myth

You can have over 13 kg (2 stone) removed by liposuction. Untrue. Although some surgeons have removed in excess of 11 ½ kg (25 lbs) with this technique, de-bulking is no longer performed, as it's dangerous. Liposuction is primarily for deposits of fat that refuse to disappear with diet and exercise and for fatty areas that drive you mad.

Breast reduction and enlargement

What is it? Breast surgery is by far the most popular cosmetic procedure in Europe. Want to go bigger, smaller, wider, higher? It can all be done. Enhancements are basically breast implants that can up your bra size from one cup size to the ridiculous four; though doctors suggest you should only ever go up two sizes.

Potential limitations: breast enlargements aren't permanent and need to be done every ten years. In the case of breast reductions, be sure to ask whether the milk ducts are cut or not, especially if one day you intend to breast-feed. Some doctors can do the operation and preserve the ducts.

What to expect: the breast enlargement operation itself is simple enough and is a bit like opening and stuffing a pillow. Scarring is minimal and exercise can be taken after only three weeks. If you're stuck for ideas on what size you'd like, throw your breasts into an uplift bra for the night and watch for reactions.

Breast reductions are a far bigger operation and involve an anchor shape being cut around your nipple (yes, the nipple is actually taken off and repositioned) and down under the breast, and then tissue is removed. At mid-operation the breast tends to look as if it has exploded, but post-op you'll have neatly defined bosoms, though with scarring that will eventually fade.

Breast uplifts are mainly for women with smaller breasts who have been hit with post-pregnancy gravity issues. The uplift involves a pulling up of the breast into a higher and

tip

Cosmetic surgery isn't for life. Breast implants have a 10 year life span and botox and collagen lips have a three to six month cycle.

perkier position. Recovery is quicker than an enhancement or reduction, as the operation is less radical.

Recovery time: two to six weeks.

Collagen lips — pumping and plumping

What is it? While fuller lips can obviously be created with the careful use of a lip liner and lip gloss, some people prefer to have a more semi-permanent plumpness to their pout with an implant, usually collagen.

Potential limitations: as sexy as this may look, be wary of exaggerating the bee-stung look. Certain celebrities have gone for lips that have ended up larger and fuller than their backside, so not a look to copy, especially if you want to look sexy. If you're tempted by lip enhancement, be aware that a horde of cowboys have set themselves up as lip specialists, and just as you wouldn't let just anybody give you root-canal work, so too should you be picky about who you let work on your lips. Potential problems include: lips that look puffy and sore, not plump, lopsided lips and lips that end up looking like they've been filled by a bicycle pump.

What to expect: the Paris lip. This is a semi-permanent treatment that uses purified bovine (that's cow to you and me) collagen, and, like normal collagen, it breaks down every three months. To create the look, a surgeon will inject collagen with a fine needle underneath the border of the upper lip to add definition. Then he will accentuate the Cupid's bow area to make a V shape (though certain surgeons don't do this and so the upper lip loses its bow shape). Finally the lower lip is treated, to balance the overall effect.

Recovery time: the overall op is painless, though you may notice a slight stinging as you're treated and some temporary swelling.

Other lip enhancement procedures use fillers known as Artecoll, and Hylaform.

Botox

What is it? Botox has been sold as the miracle beauty treatment of the decade. Worried about getting old, hate your frown lines, want to get rid of your stern look and appear calm when you're raging inside? Well, Botox is apparently the answer. This 'miracle treatment' has come about because we've basically become a society obsessed with looking young. This is particularly bad news is you're a female, because we rely on the hormone oestrogen. When we have a good supply of this hormone, skin remains soft, supple, healthy and resilient but unfortunately, as oestrogen levels start to decrease at the onset of peri-menopause (the bit before menopause, around your mid-thirties) skin rapidly starts losing its vitality and

tip

If surgery's not for you, think about a cheat's guide to getting the body you want. Look for bras that lift and squeeze, knickers that push upwards, lipsticks that plump and face gels that tighten.

firmness. From your forties onwards, the fine skin under the eyes will also lose its tautness and smoothness, and cause a bagging look. From 50, the elastin fibres that support the skin decline dramatically, and accelerate drooping and sagging around the cheeks.

Potential limitations: bearing all this in mind it's little wonder so many women have flocked to Botox clinics for a helping hand. Botox, or rather botulinum toxin, as you might have heard, is a form of botulism and poisonous to the body in large quantities. It's this that is injected in teeny amounts into the muscle in your forehead to give you a smoother look (also used for migraine treatments and sweating, see Chapter 6).

What to expect: once there, the Botox works by literally paralysing the muscles in the forehead so when you try to frown you can't, meaning you're wrinkle-free. It's great for a youthful look albeit one devoid of expression! The bad news is no one yet knows the long-term consequences of having three shots a year injected into your head (that's over 30 doses in ten years). Specialists say people shouldn't worry, as the toxin is not injected into the bloodstream, but the truth is only time will tell.

Recovery time: the treatment takes about four days to work effectively.

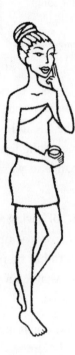

The new fillers

Botox may work for the upper areas of your face, but it's not so hot for the lower reaches, simply because no one wants to walk around with a mouth that won't move. While fat and collagen have long been used to plump up the face, the fact remains that fat and collagen don't last when injected into the face. Plus collagen can trigger an allergic reaction. These new fillers are said to be cheaper and longer-lasting but, as yet, many have not been 100 per cent approved for use in many countries.

Perlane: is a transparent gel based on hyaluronic acid, which works like collagen. It is injected into the lips and cheeks to plump them out for a more youthful appearance. It lasts for about a year, unlike collagen, which lasts around three months.

Restylane: is bacteria synthesised into acid form. Good for upper lips, nose folds and lip plumping.

Hylaform: another type of synthesised acid, and also good for nasal folds and lips. Said to be excellent for natural-looking results and long-lasting effects.

Artecoll: a combination of collagen and plastic. Good for scars and deep creases, as the plastic remains in the skin and eventually the body deposits its own collagen over it, once the injected collagen has gone. Potential pitfalls are the fact that it is permanent and can go wrong if it's over-applied. Not good for lips.

Silicone: liquid droplets that are good for lips, nasal folds and frown lines. It's another permanent technique but it can cause inflammation and/or nodules to appear. Long-term problems with silicone are also known.

Nose job/rhinoplasty

What is it? Nose reshaping is in the top ten of the most performed cosmetic procedures in Europe and the US and is known as a rhinoplasty. The operation is one of the few that can make a radical and fairly instant change to your face.

Potential limitations: if you've always dreamed of having a perfect nose, doctors warn that you should lower your expectations and go for a nose that suits you, rather than choose someone else's. Also, be realistic about what a new nose will do for you, or you'll end up disappointed.

What to expect: the operation itself takes about one hour to perform, during which the nasal cartilage is removed and reshaped within the nasal cavity. It sounds a big operation and it is, so expect two black eyes and a puffy nose for a while.

Recovery time: the good news is, make-up can be worn by the third day and you'll only have to stay in hospital for a night.

myth

The nose crumbles after a nose job. Untrue. This is one of those myths perpetuated by a certain famous celebrity who has had so many nose jobs his nasal cavity has now caved in. The good news is it won't happen to you unless you decide to have more than your fair share of operations.

Perfect skin

We all love baby skin, simply because it's smooth, plump, wrinkle-free and hasn't yet been ravaged by daily living, the remnants of teenage spots and bad habits. However, if your skin has, don't despair; there's now a multitude of beauty procedures that can smooth out/laser/peel and blast your skin into shape.

Peels

Acid face peels work by lifting off the top layer of dead skin cells, a process that can be achieved just as efficiently with some exfoliating (see Chapter 1).

Most over-the-counter beauty products contain some sort of peeling ingredient: think AHAs (alpha hydroxy acids), fruit acids and glycolic acid, which help get rid of dead skin cells. However, the peels used by beauty therapists and doctors tend to be more powerful and aggressive;

meaning a deeper peel, which will eventually reveal fresher-looking skin underneath.

Sandblasting, aka microdermabrasion

This is something that has to be done in a salon by a trained professional. The process involves the problem area of your face literally being blasted by fine sand-like crystals at high speed. This process removes dead skin cells, smoothes out fine lines and helps decrease the appearance of acne scars. If done properly, microdermabrasion shouldn't hurt, but it will leave your skin feeling very tender – one therapist noted that after your first treatment you should aim to stay in all weekend, as your skin will be sore and you may look as if you have chickenpox! Treatment can take from around 40 minutes to an hour and is usually performed as a course of ten.

It's worth noting that though microdermabrasion works, it will not get rid of deep scars, sort out spots or deal with problems such as sun-damaged skin, broken veins and moles. Plus, it should not be performed if you have sunburnt skin, sensitive skin or an open wound.

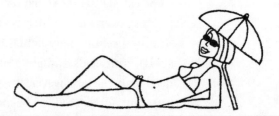

20 ways to avoid surgery and still look like Barbie

1 Do facial exercises

Use it or lose it applies to every muscle in your body, including your face. If you want to avoid Botox, facials and surgery, exercise your face for ten minutes every day. You can do this the lazy way by having a good laugh with friends, or stand in front of your mirror and grin and relax ten times; raise and lower your eyebrows ten times; and then puff your cheeks up with air and release.

2 Wear the right bra

Studies show 75 per cent of us don't wear the correct bra and cup size, which means in some cases we're aiding gravity, and in others we're not making the most of our assets. To get the shape you want, get measured at a shop, and try on a variety of bras. With uplifts, balconies, and minimisers even large breasts can be made small and small breasts made huge!

3 Draw bigger lips

Top make-up tip: use a lip liner that matches your lip colour to draw just outside your natural lip line, and then make it connect at the corners of your lip and gently fill in. The aim is to plump up your pout as naturally as possible.

4 Use some gloss

Perfect your pout by adding a dollop of lip gloss to the centre of your lower lip. This not only plumps the lip out, but also makes your lips appear fuller and sexier. For a longer-lasting look, invest in one of the many volumising lip treatments, usually known as lip plumps and pulps. These have ingredients that literally make your lips look as if they have had the collagen injection.

5 Avoid your wrinkles

As in avoid when you're putting on your make-up. Filling the creases with foundation and powder just causes them to crinkle when you smile, and draws attention to them.

6 Bite a lemon

One beauty editor swears that the best way to get sexy, pouty lips before going out at night is to bite on a lemon while you're getting ready. Cheaper than collagen by far.

7 Choose your lipstick carefully

Dark colours and matt lipsticks make lips look thinner and drier. Stick to gloss shades closer to your natural colour or something that has added shimmer to accentuate your lips.

8 Do leg lifts instead of lipo

Want thin thighs but can't afford liposuction? Easy, do some lunges; they're top of the class for bum and thigh toning. The secret lies in the fact they simultaneously tone the thighs and bum. Stand with your feet slightly apart, hold your tummy in and take a big step forward (i.e. lunge). As the front foot lands, bend the front knee so that your hips drop between your feet and your back knee goes down. Then push back to your starting position. Do three sets of 15–20 repetitions alternating between legs.

9 Step up for collagen production

As in join a step class or do some other kind of aerobic exercise. Studies show there is a measurable improvement in the elasticity of skin amongst people who exercise and raise their heartbeat more than three times a week. Skin looks younger, firmer, brighter and suppler and stays this way for longer.

10 Squat to get the bottom you want

Stand with your feet slightly wider than shoulder width. Imagine you're about to sit on a chair, and, keeping your stomach pulled in and your back straight, literally squat down. Keep the knees in line with your toes at all times. Slowly return to the start position and repeat.
Do two sets of 15–20 repeats.

11 Cheat your way to a flat tummy

For a no-effort technique: try a body wrap at a beauty salon. Most work on a firming, exfoliating and trussing-you-up-in-cling-film basis. Although inches lost are from water and not fat, the effect usually lasts for about five days.

12 Stand tall

The key to looking long and lean is good posture. Imagine that there's a string pulling you up from the centre of your head. This way your back will be in the right position, your stomach will be supported and you'll look half a stone lighter immediately.

13 Beat the bloat

For a flat stomach it's essential to look at the foods you're eating. Retaining water and having gas in your stomach will sabotage your chances of getting a six-pack look. To help yourself, avoid eating too many starchy carbohydrates – potatoes, rice, bread and pasta – at night; eat them at lunchtime instead. This is because simple carbohydrates are stored mostly as fat at night.

14 Reduce your stress levels

If you eat too fast, you won't chew food properly, and you'll end up washing your food down and/or swallowing too much air which will then cause a tummy as round as a basketball.

15 Have a massage

Apart from ironing out hunched shoulders and making your body feel suppler, massages have a more powerful health message to pummel home. Recent medical research shows that apart from diminishing aches and pains, massage can boost circulation, decrease levels of stress hormones, balance the nervous system, and stimulate the nerves that supply blood to the internal organs; leaving you with less tension and anxiety in your body and helping you to look and feel younger.

16 Visit the optician

Avoid those fine lines and the need for Botox by not only wearing sunglasses to erase the sun's glare but also making sure you get your eyes checked. The Royal National Institute for the Blind estimates 27.5 million people should be having an eye test each year, but only 15 million are, which means 12.5 million are missing out. If you can't see properly, you're more likely to adopt a squinty-eyed look.

17 Take your vitamins

For those who can't be bothered to rub cream into their face, never mind have surgery, but still want to look fabulous for life, work on the internal side and take some vitamins and minerals for the whole body:

B vitamins: essential for healthy skin and hair.

Vitamin D: for healthy bones and hair.

Vitamin E: a must for healthy skin.

Iron: for energy.

Calcium: for bones and teeth.

Vitamin C: for a healthy immune system.

18 Have sex regularly

Use it or lose it is the maxim for staying young both mentally and physically. Have sex at least once a week and you'll not only look better but also feel better and give yourself a workout equivalent to going to the gym.

19 Do some exercise

Yes, this old chestnut again, but a guaranteed way of looking and feeling younger for life. If gym life is not for you, consider becoming more active. Walk more, climb steps, run for the bus, even go out dancing. It will keep your muscles firm and lean, and in turn will help you feel young.

20 Revive your skin

Do some rigorous body brushing. Brush upwards and towards the heart to not only exfoliate your entire body but also to expel nasties, such as toxins, and improve circulation so your skin takes on a fabulous, sexy, youthful glow.

chapter 5
The icky bits

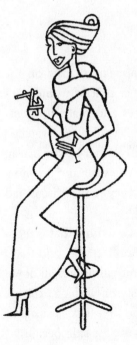

Beauty, unfortunately, is not just about making the most of your gorgeous bits. While it's fun to perfect your pout, experiment with face creams, eye masks and body lotions, the fact remains there are icky bits to be dealt with; bits that need a serious beauty MOT, and on a fairly constant basis. Of course, you may be a surface kind of chick. Someone who can only be bothered to perfect the parts everyone can see; a Band-aid kind of girl, who is quite happy to hide her personal nasties under clothes, make-up and sarongs. However, ignore these bits at your peril. Bad habits will eventually show up on your body and skin. Slovenly beauty routines will have your body sliding downwards and outwards, and buying expensive creams to cover up the fact that your favourite meal is a bag of crisps will not save you from skin the texture of a crisp bag. Save yourself now: here's how.

What's up with your skin?

By now you should have cottoned on that beauty is more than skin-deep, but that's no consolation if your skin is suddenly puckering and dimpling and growing things you'd rather not see. Here's how to look good and feel good about your skin glitches.

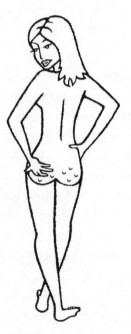

Cellulite

It resembles dimply orange peel, appears mainly on the thighs and bottom and affects 85 per cent of women. It's also the stuff that beauty magazines and make-up companies go into a mass frenzy about. If you've ever watched someone pummelling their backside with a bristly brush, buying botty cream as expensive as a new car and downing gallons of water, you can guarantee they've just discovered they have cellulite.

The good news is cellulite is not something that is inexplicable or hard to get your head round. It's fat, and that's all there is to it. The reason it becomes dimply is all down to a lack of the male hormone testosterone, which explains why lardy boys don't get it – seeing as they have lashings of the stuff. Testosterone is important for the skin because it strengthens collagen, the very fibre that keeps skin taut and firm. Collagen also helps hold fat cells together – without it things literally collapse. When testosterone depletes, and you don't do any exercise to keep the skin firm, the fat cells lose their round shape and become pointy. Fat then fills the shape, giving you that dimply look.

Zap your cellulite by ...

Doing some exercise

This is the number-one way to beat cellulite. It keeps the body's fat levels down and helps keep skin firm and taut. Make sure you do 30 to 40 minutes of exercise three to four times a week. Ensure it includes cardiovascular work, such as power-walking, running or cycling, and weights, such as free weights. Pilates and yoga will also help, though don't make this your only source of exercise. Target your bottom with:

The lunge: this exercise is top of its class for bum and thigh toning. Its secret lies in the fact that it simultaneously tones the thighs and bum. Stand with your feet slightly apart, hold your tummy in and lunge (take a big step) forward. As the front foot lands, bend the front knee so that your hips drop between your feet and your back knee goes down. Then push back to your starting position.

tip

Cellulite busting is easier than you think. It's fat so exercise it away with high intensity work-outs, for an hour three times a week.

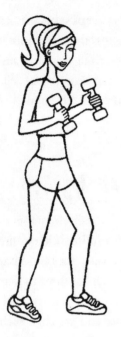

Do three sets of 15–20 repetitions alternating between legs.

The static lunge: this is very similar to the above, the only difference being that once you have lunged forward you stay in position and move up and down in a vertical movement. Go down until the knee is a few centimetres off the floor, then come up.

Do three sets of 15–20 repetitions on each leg.

The squat: great for a firm bottom. Stand with your feet slightly wider than shoulder width. Imagine you're about to sit on a chair and, keeping your stomach pulled in and your back straight, squat down. Keep the knees in line with your toes at all times. Slowly return to the start position and repeat.

Do two sets of 15–20 reps.

Kneeling kick back: get down on all fours, and with your back straight pull your stomach muscles in. Raise and bend

myth

Cellulite is the result of toxin build-up from a bad diet, coffee and smoking. Untrue. Cellulite is fat and that's all there is to it. Which is why your unhealthiest mate can have skin as smooth as a baby's bottom and still live the party life.

one leg at a 90-degree angle, then lower the leg back to just above the floor and repeat 15–20 times; swap legs and repeat.

Investing in cellulite treatments

Cellulite creams don't work, but one technique, which has been proven to work by clinical trials, is endermologie. This is a deep-tissue massage that uses a machine to pummel your cells back into shape. As for creams, they can improve the outer layers of skin so use one with active ingredients that are known to help. Try those that contain escin, horse chestnut tree extract, and good old aloe vera, available from all chemists. These stimulate the blood flow in the skin.

Having a massage

Recent medical research from Middlesex University Hospital, London shows that apart from diminishing aches and pains, massage can boost circulation and stimulate the nerves that supply blood to the internal organs. All of which is good news for you and bad news for cellulite.

Eating the right foods

Reducing the level of fat in your diet is key. Aim for foods rich in omega 3 and 6 fatty acids (EFAs). These not only regulate the speed at which fat is released into the body but also research shows they have a definite anti-cellulite effect.

EFAs are found in oily fish, especially salmon and tuna, flaxseeds, linseeds and nuts. Ensure you eat oily fish at least twice a week or take a supplement.

Upping your intake of antioxidants

These help eradicate free radicals – naturally occurring rogue molecules that also damage the shape of fat cells. Antioxidants can be found in onions, cloves and garlic and vitamins A, C and E, plus the minerals selenium, zinc and manganese.

Buying a body brush

Dry skin brushing won't rid your body of cellulite but it will help with the overall look of your skin as it aids lymph drainage and helps your skin to look less puffy and sallow. Work the brush in movements towards your heart, focusing on moving up the legs in long sweeping strokes.

tip

If you've ended up looking like a slice of streaky bacon, help yourself by using a daily body scrub to help the tan to fade and then even up the stripes with a bronzing powder.

Stretch marks

These are those lovely track lines that traverse your belly, back, thighs, arms or anywhere where your body has suddenly changed shape. In reality these purple, white and red marks are breakdowns in the elastic fibres of the skin, which usually occur when the skin has been stretched excessively (think pregnancy, weight gain, puberty). Sadly there is no miracle cure, but if you keep them well moisturised with aloe vera or normal body oil or lotion, they will eventually fade and be noticeable only to you.

If you loathe them beyond belief, there are two treatments available to zap them:

Futur-Tec Skin Regeneration System: an ultrasound and vacuum therapy, which stimulates blood flow and leaves stretch marks smoother and less noticeable. It's a non-invasive procedure that leaves a slight tingling sensation. It's not a quick fix: you need between six and ten sessions.

ERP (electroridopuncture) technology: helps repair stretch marks by boosting collagen and elastin and helping with repigmentation – stretch marks tend to look paler than the surrounding skin. You'll need three treatments to notice a major difference.

Other than the above, don't stress about stretch marks. Everyone has them, especially guys, who usually get them as a result of the growth spurt at puberty.

tip

Use Aloe Vera, body oil and massage oil to help stretch marks fade.

Moles and beauty spots

A genetic throwback to one of your relatives, moles usually appear during childhood. If you're predisposed to them, you'll usually end up with around ten to 20 in varying sizes and places (smaller ones are usually found on the face and have become known as beauty spots).

Moles naturally occur in areas of the skin where there is a heavy amount of pigmentation (melanin) and begin as flat brown spots that become raised and then fade. The majority of moles are harmless and can be removed; though if you go down this route you should expect a certain amount of scarring.

One mole in a million becomes a melanoma – skin cancer – and this is the direct result of sun damage. If you have a mole that suddenly grows in size, becomes itchy, changes colour, bleeds or has ragged edges, see your doctor as soon as possible.

myth

You can get cancer if you pluck hairs in moles. Untrue. However hairy moles should be trimmed, not plucked, as this leaves the mole open to bacteria and possible infection.

Sun damage

Forget sunburn, long-term sun damage manifests itself as brown pigmentation marks, moles and wrinkly, papery skin. The bad news is: nothing, not even a mega-expensive face cream, will ward off these wrinkles and discolouring.

If you have them, your best bet is a cover-up with make-up and moisturiser to make your skin retain its hydration levels.

The best cure for sun-damaged skin is prevention. To maintain your looks and still go out in the sun:

- Always wear a sunscreen in the sun, and even on cloudy summer days, with a protection factor of no less than SPF 15. Reapply every two hours and don't be fooled into thinking you can decrease the protection factor as the time goes on. The skin does not become resilient to ultraviolet rays.
- Don't use tanning booths/sunbeds. Contrary to popular belief the UVA rays they use are not harmless and can cause deeper damage to the skin. A 10-minute roast on a bed equals an entire day without sunscreen on the beach.
- Wear sunscreen even if you're under a shaded umbrella, as pavement, sand and water all reflect 85 per cent of the sun's rays, and a T-shirt gives you only about a factor 6–8 protection level – and that's just on the covered-up bits.
- Wear a very high factor on your sun-damaged bits, as they are more vulnerable to the sun.

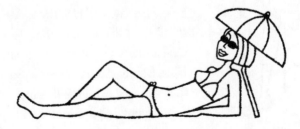

What's up with your body?

There's having a good time that is good for you and then there's having a good time that is bad for you, and you probably don't need me to tell you which habits are the unhealthy ones. Even if you don't care a hoot about your health, it's worth bearing in mind that too many hedonistic nights equals a face that even your mother won't love. To look gorgeous, act bad and still party, here's how to keep your looks in shape.

Boozing

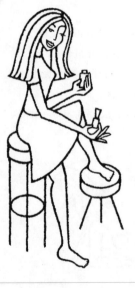

While a glass of wine has been proven to be good for your heart, it's not always great for your looks. This is because alcohol can make you look older, as it dehydrates the body's main organs and decreases the elasticity of the skin, causing it to age faster, become more wrinkled and basically makes you look as if you have been dragged through a hedge backwards. Healthy guidelines suggest that women should not drink more than 14 units of alcohol per week. One unit is equivalent to a small glass of low-strength wine, a single short or half a pint of lager, but bear in mind that stronger drinks will contain more units of alcohol.

To maintain your looks while you party make sure you:

- Don't order double measures and mix your drinks with sugar-laden colas.
- Drink double the amount of water for every drink you swallow.
- Don't go over your weekly limit (14 units).
- Eat before you start drinking – you'll drink less and consume fewer calories, plus you won't wake up with a hangover face.
- Avoid cocktails, as there can be as many as three units in one glass.
- To preserve your looks start with some preventative measures. Antioxidants are particularly apt at fighting off alcohol damage and protecting your liver. They also stop your brain cells being killed off by weekend binges. Found in green leafy vegetables and fruit. Aim to get ample amounts of vitamins A, C and E in the days before a big night out.

tip

Don't overscrutinise your body. If you peer at yourself too closely you're bound to find weird bumps and lumps. The good news is no-one will ever know they are there but you (unless of course you point them out).

To look gorgeous the morning after

- Drink water; that might seem obvious but you need to down at least 2 litres ($3\frac{1}{2}$ pints) to overcome dehydration and mind-numbing headaches.
- Avoid a carbohydrate and fat binge – it will make you sleepy and lethargic.
- Graze, don't stuff your face – eat something small every few hours for maximum energy.
- Avoid the latte – stick to fruit juices instead for maximum energy.
- Eat live yoghurt to combat post-party breath.

- Take the herbal aid artichoke and milk thistle the night before to help aid digestion. You can try anything with extract of artichoke and milk thistle.
- Beat upset tummies with indigestion tablets – excellent if you've overindulged all night.
- Finally take a recovery drink. This is a carbonated, vitamin-enriched powder you mix with water that's designed to help you feel fine the morning after.
- Moisturise your face to avoid the dehydrating effects of alcohol.
- Place cucumber slices on your eyes and use eye drops to avoid red, hard-to-open eyes.
- Exfoliate at night to help your skin get rid of all the alcohol toxins it's been excreting all day.
- Get an early night but make sure you get up at your usual time so your body clock doesn't go haywire.

Smoking — it kills your looks

We all know smoking kills and that smoking-related diseases are on the increase, but did you also know smoking will kill your looks? Yup, the 4,000 chemicals in just one cigarette will give you grey sallow skin (all that smoke nestling around your cheekbones), and bad breath. It will also deepen facial lines around your eyes and mouth, dehydrate your skin and make you age faster. If that wasn't enough, it will make your hair stink and your hands yellow. Here's how:

It will make your skin look grey

To stay healthy your skin relies on a healthy blood supply to pump away beneath the skin. Nicotine, unfortunately, constricts blood vessels, starving the skin of vital oxygen.

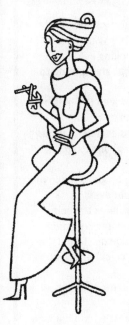

It gives you bad breath

Smoking dries out the membranes inside your mouth, which are responsible for producing saliva. With no saliva to kill off bacteria regularly you're asking for some deadly halitosis. The truth is most smokers have bad breath (even if they suck extra-strong mints) because the chemicals from each puff naturally linger in their mouths producing some very pungent and nasty smells.

It will kill your megawatt smile

Studies show smoking can also give you gum disease: gingivitis, also known as inflammation of the gums, can set in because smoking eats away at your mouth's defence mechanism.

It will make you snore like a pig

Not a beauty problem, but it will ruin your beauty-goddess image in bed.

It will make you look 50 when you're 30 years old

Smoking in particular is bad news in the ageing stakes, as cigarettes load the body with free radicals (molecules

Beauty tips for smoking girls

- Massage your face daily – use your fingertips and gently rub the skin in small clockwise circles. This will increase blood flow to your face and stop you looking ashen.
- Exfoliate regularly to help the toxins that are fighting to get out of your skin.
- Consider using a daily protection cream with SPF in it, as this will help protect the skin from smoke.
- Boost your skin growth with a healthy diet (see Chapters 3 and 6), regular face masks (see Chapter 7) and exercise. All will help get rid of your smoker's face.
- Don't forget the eye cream, as smoking tends to make you squint to avoid the smoke getting in your eyes.
- Drink plenty of water, as smoking dehydrates the body.
- Invest in a facial – it will give your skin instant radiance.
- Don't cake on the make-up. Too much powder, foundation and concealer will just make your face 'crack' when you start puffing away.
- To get rid of yellowing fingers, soak your digits in lemon juice and then moisturise.
- For a radiant glow when you've really partied too hard, go for shimmer to lift your skin. Aim for upper eyelids and cheekbones, and then gloss your lips. Avoid heavy panda-style eyes and dark matt lipsticks.

which destroy healthy cells in the body), dehydrate the skin, create fine wrinkles and give you lung and bronchial problems. The good news is: give up and within eight hours levels of poisonous carbon monoxide in your blood will drop to normal. Within two days your chances of a heart attack decrease and within a year premature wrinkling decreases.

What's up with your insides?

You can sometimes be the healthiest person in the world and still find that your insides are not playing the game. This of course has all kinds of implications for your looks. Stuffed-up insides, food allergies, too much partying can all play havoc with your internal detox system. If your skin, hair and body need a jump-start, take a look at what you can do from the inside out.

Colonic irrigation

A little stuffed up? Well, here's something that you can do in the name of beauty: colonic irrigation, or colonic therapy, is the human equivalent of calling the plumber in, and

tip

Red bumps on your upper arms are a form of dermatitis caused by hair follicles clogged with oil and dead skin. Don't over-scrub, but improve the circulation to the upper arms – do push ups and triceps dips – and then use a body lotion with AHA's (alpha hydroxy acids) to help the skin exfoliate and repair itself.

whether it has you cringing in horror or jumping for joy, devotees say it's a marvellous way to feel full of plenty of energy and have glowingly fresh skin.

Despite what you're thinking, a colonic is a painless procedure whereby a small (and we're talking small) plastic tube is inserted into your bottom so that water can be pumped in to flush out your blocked-up waste and toxins. On the whole, however, it's worth noting that doctors are against this treatment because they fear the insertion of the tube carries a risk, albeit very, very low, of perforating the bowel; therapists say this is impossible, if you visit a trained professional.

myth

Colonics can uncover all kinds of nasties in your gut. Untrue. If you're worried about the pain and/or possible bizarre finds in your waste, it's worth noting that, despite the urban myths, colonic therapy won't unload any scary objects, long-lost toys, last year's Xmas dinner or any weird stuff from your gut. All that comes out is normal waste and undigested food with the help of the water and a gentle external massage around the colon.

Detoxing — what goes in, comes out

Spring-cleaning your system, or detoxing, is where you pare your diet down to raw and very healthy foods for a short period of time in order to rid the body of toxins, which slow your system down and give you bad skin and lank hair.

These toxins come from a variety of external sources such as certain fatty foods, cigarettes, alcohol, stress, anxiety and environmental pollutants. On the beauty front they ruin your looks, as they tend to act like poison. The aim of a detox is, therefore, to eliminate all beauty nasties by cleansing the intestinal tract, i.e. working from the inside out.

The good news is: these days a detox diet doesn't mean fasting for days, eating copious amounts of brown rice, and/or denying yourself everything you like. In fact you should avoid following a rigorous regime of denial, as this can actually be more harmful to the body. It releases too many toxins too quickly and can leave you feeling nauseous with bad breath, terrible skin and a killer headache.

The detox diet

Before you start a detox, ease yourself into the cleansing programme gradually or else your body will retaliate horribly (think flatulence and spots).

In the run-up, cut down on the above toxin-releasing foods, especially coffee, so you don't suffer withdrawal symptoms during the detox. Then aim to follow a low-fat diet, rich in vegetables and fruit. This is also the time to start upping your intake of water – essential for a successful detox.

The detox rules

1. Remember to take things easy, as you'll begin to feel tired as the detox process starts to work.
2. Drink lots of water – at least 2 litres (3½ pints) a day – to stop dehydration and speed up the cleansing process.
3. Never detox if you are pregnant, breastfeeding, diabetic, on medication, have kidney or liver problems or are ill.

To detox, cut out ...

Coffee and tea: five to six cups a day can lead to caffeine toxicity, which results in restlessness, dry skin and tiredness.

Alcohol: this is extremely toxic and can lead to liver damage, heart strain and dehydration.

Salt: this aids dehydration and causes bloating.

Sugar: this accelerates mood swings and headaches.

Dairy: these are mucus-forming foods, which release toxins that cause sinus problems and skin complaints.

The weekend detox

Start every day with a glass of warm water and lemon juice to flush your system out.

Breakfast: eat as much fresh fruit as you like – grapes, apples and melon are a good choice, though bananas tend to be too starchy and oranges too acidic. Add live bio yoghurt. For a drink, make yourself a pot of herbal tea or opt for fruit juice. Fruit is an excellent start to the day, as it helps to activate the liver – the body's main cleansing organ – and stimulates the bowel. It also gives you all the essential vitamins and minerals you need. The live bio yoghurt will help to cleanse and balance the good and bad bacteria in your gut.

tip

For smooth skin on your upper arms – exercise your arms to maintain a healthy blood flow to the area. Improved circulation equals improved skin.

Lunch: make a salad with mixed raw vegetables. Use olive oil on the salad to help you digest it. The enzymes in the raw vegetables will boost your metabolism and give you some energy, while the fibre will speed up the cleansing process.

Snacks: nibble on grated carrots or apple slices, and/or drink plenty of water – it sounds harsh and dull, but remember, you're doing this for only a few days.

Dinner: aim to have your last meal of the day before 8 p.m., as this gives you plenty of time to digest food before going to sleep. Though raw is best, if you can't face another salad, lightly steam some fresh vegetables, or stir-fry them in a wok and season to taste.

Days two and three

Stick to the above diet but add 115 g (4 oz) of poached or grilled fish, and some short-grain brown rice to your steamed vegetables at dinner.

Ten ways to make the detox last

1. Eat five servings of fruit and vegetables a day.
2. Drink at least 8–12 glasses of water a day.
3. Cut down on coffee.
4. Eat lean meats, and fish in preference to red meat.
5. Exercise for at least 20 minutes every day (even if it's just a walk to the shops).
6. Learn to relax and de-stress.
7. Don't eat late at night.
8. Take an antioxidant.
9. Stop smoking – the perfect way to stop toxins entering your body.
10. Drink less alcohol – one or two small drinks a day is fine, but don't go over your units per week, as this will ruin the effects of the detox on your system.

Reactions to detoxing

During the detox diet there may be some side effects:

- Some people find themselves with a headache. This is triggered by the release of toxins from the body. If it is severe or won't go away, you are probably being too strict with your diet, and need to eat and drink more.
- Enhance the effects by taking care of your skin. It's one of the biggest organs of toxin elimination, and skin brushing will help stimulate the lymphatic system.
- Others find they have a bad taste in their mouth; again this is caused by toxins being expelled. A good tip is to rinse your mouth with hot water and lemon juice and/or scrape your tongue with a teaspoon.
- If you get an outbreak of spots or your skin becomes dry, don't panic, this is only a temporary reaction.
- You may also feel more tired than you did before the detox; this occurs because your body is using up energy to expel waste from your system. Don't reach for a coffee, just curl up and relax – it won't last beyond 24 hours.

20 ways
to deal with horrible
beauty moments

1 Blink away the redness
Lose the bloodshot eyes fast by using eye-drops that contain naphazoline; they will constrict the eye veins and help you lose the drunken wino look.

2 Scrub your face
Partying all night is bad news for your skin. as it makes dead skin cells stick to it giving you a sallow slept-in-a-hedge look. Exfoliate with a face cloth for a more radiant look.

3 Cool your cheeks
Red, blotchy hangover skin? Soak a face cloth in tepid water and lay it over the face for five to ten minutes. It will alleviate redness and your headache.

4 Eat some strawberries
They contain masses of vitamin C – a potent skin brightener, and essential for a healthy glow.

5 Fill up on greens
A vitamin-rich plant-based diet keeps your skin looking great and your hair glossy, even if you skip the sleep and overindulge. Eat broccoli, romaine lettuce and green leafy vegetables as often as possible.

6 Moisturise even more
Especially when you're hungover and it's the change of season. To get rough skin smooth, hydrate with a rich moisturiser every evening for four nights and then go back to your normal routine.

7 Clean your teeth
A whiter smile can double your glow. Plus white teeth will not only make you appear healthier but will also light up your look. Use whitening toothpastes to get rid of surface stains, see your dentist for deeper ones and use a red lip gloss to show off your clean teeth.

8 Think about your breath

Forget the gum, chew parsley, as it's heaped full of chlorophyll, which will zap halitosis fast. Chew one sprig until you can't bear it any longer.

9 Put your feet first

A much-avoided area of the body. If your tootsies pong a little too strongly, be sure to wear different shoes every other day – otherwise odour will build up in your shoes. Also, spray feet with a deodorant and sprinkle with talc to help soak up the sweat.

10 Mash a banana into your hair

If your hair is rebelling at the copious amounts of products you've piled into it, help rehydrate it with a banana. Mash up a ripe one and massage into your scalp. Leave it for ten minutes and then rinse out.

11 Use perfume on spots

Stuck for some spot help? If you're desperate, you can use perfume, as it contains alcohol. Don't spray directly, put some on your clean finger, dab on, let it dry and apply concealer to cover up.

12 Rub salt into your flaky lips

Exfoliate dry, flaky lips with rock salt (don't rub too hard and break the skin), rinse off and apply lip salve to gloss your lips and moisturise.

13 Always keep Vaseline in your bag

It's the number-one beauty must-have and perfect to avoid morning-after horrors. It can be used as a cleanser and a moisturiser, and if you're stuck without your make-up bag just rub some into the palm of your hand until it liquefies, and then apply to your face.

14 Banish the effects of 20 a day

Stock up on vitamin C, as this is heavily depleted when you smoke, and a lack of it not only leaves your skin looking grey and your hair ashen but also weakens your immune system, leaving you susceptible to mouth ulcers and colds.

15 Beware of rashes

If you've woken up with a nasty stubble rash across your chin, soothe it with some calamine lotion (the stuff your mum used to put on chickenpox). If you're going out, apply some emulsifying cream, available from your chemist. This sits on the skin and protects the raw area. Avoid make-up until the area is less raw.

16 Alleviate puffiness

Get the good old cucumber out, and this time layer slices across your face, concentrating on the areas that look the puffiest. Ten minutes of relaxing with slices will leave skin refreshed and less bloated.

17 Deflate the bags under your eyes

Be careful what you use around the eyes as the skin here is very thin and sensitive. If you have bigger luggage here than in an aircraft's hold, simply soak two cotton-wool pads in cold water, pat off excess water and lay over the eyes. This will tighten the skin and leave it less baggy.

18 Think dewy, not matte

Especially if you're suffering from a serious hangover, as you're likely to be sweating toxins. Creamy-based make-up looks more natural and goes on more easily, while matt make-up tends to sit on the skin emphasising your previous heavy night.

19 Don't overdo the perfume

Apart from making you feel ill, it won't help that headache. If you've overindulged, keep your perfume simple. Stick to essential oils: grapefruit for energy, mint to wake you up and eucalyptus to clear your head and make you feel cleansed.

20 Avoid perfection

The tried-too-hard look will give you away in an instant. Morning-after make-up should be relaxed and easy. Apply a gloss stain with your fingers, keep hair unstructured and tousled, and don't go for the full make-up look. Think sunglasses over mascara and liner.

chapter 6
Disaster zone

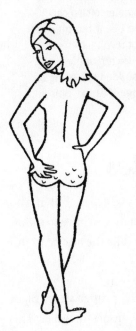

So you did everything right. You drank your 2 litres (3½ pints) of water, made yourself go to bed at 11 p.m., took off your make-up before you hit the pillow and even thought about giving up smoking and joining a gym. So why are you looking at a beauty disaster in the mirror? How come your face is dotted with spots, your hair is standing on end and dark circles are navigating your eyes? Worse still, why are people telling you look tired/peaky and grey?

Even if you know where you went wrong – too much sun, too much booze, too little sleep – a beauty disaster is bad news for even the laziest girl. Apart from being a major self-esteem blow, walking around with sweat patches under your arms, excess body hair sprouting from your bits, red, peeling skin and bad breath is something even your best friend is unlikely to put up with on a long-term basis.

Good thing then that this chapter can offer you instant help in rebuilding the disaster zone that is your body. Follow it carefully, if you want to achieve the natural beauty look successfully without looking too wild and rugged.

myth

You can cover up any beauty disaster. Untrue. Sadly, some beauty glitches are too big and too obvious to slap concealer over, and, in some cases, shouldn't be attempted at home. If your face is displaying signs of revolt – think soreness, weeping wounds and itchiness – do not apply anything over it. The same goes for a sudden sprouting of hair, a weird vein or skin that's shearing off like an onion!

The disaster rules

OK, you want to solve your beauty glitches, but if you really truly want to zap them completely you have to follow certain rules for a week, and not just take the advice in this chapter and ignore the obvious:

Rule one, get some sleep: this means proper sleep. Eight hours' worth each night, that's 56 hours a week. This

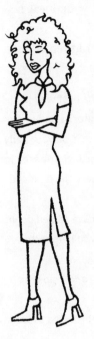

doesn't mean five hours during the week and 31 hours over the weekend.

Rule two, drink more water: again this doesn't mean mix your wine with sparkling water, down 2 litres (3½ pints) of the stuff and then congratulate yourself on your new-found love of water.

Rule three, get some exercise: walking to the TV set doesn't count. Walking to work does.

Rule four, eat all food groups: that's not choccie biscuits, crisps, toast and peanut butter with an odd pizza thrown in, but three proper meals a day with veggies that still look like vegetables.

Rule five, see your doctor asap: if your beauty glitch looks disastrous. Clues: it's open, sore, falling out, itchy, spreading or painful.

The body blips

Sunburn

OK, I won't go into the obvious lecture on the sun, skin cancer and ageing, because if you've overdone the tan, you'll know it and probably be suffering for it. Apart from feeling an excruciating skin-peeling-like pain, it's likely you also resemble a tandoori dish from your local take-away.

To help with the soreness, your mum's old remedies are the best.

1. A cool compress laid over your burnt bits is the best way to deal with immediate pain. Soak a towel in water at body-temperature, not ice-cold, and wring out. Place it on your body. If you have burnt your body badly, see your local pharmacist for a hydrocortisone cream that can help take away the pain and soothe the skin.
2. A soothing balm on sunburnt skin *after* you have cooled down and taken the initial pain away is a good way to help restore the skin. Try aloe vera.
3. Take an aspirin or ibuprofen to block the pain and help with skin inflammation.
4. Drink lots of water; the chances are you're dehydrated as well.

Sweating

There are certain situations where you're going to sweat naturally a lot; for example, when it's 75 degrees outside, when you've been working out, when your period is due and when you're wearing a variety of man-made fibres in August. (However, if you're sweating and everyone else is complaining of the cold you need to get checked out by your doctor for hormonal imbalances and diabetes.) After trying the obvious, if you still smell like yesterday's old socks, you can consider keyhole surgery called endoscopic thoracic sympathicotomy, a permanent procedure that involves severing nerves to stop the nervous system sending signals to the sweat glands. Alternatively, try Botox, which is semi-permanent. Botox is 99 per cent effective for sweating problems, as the toxin is injected into the armpit to inhibit sweat production under the arm. Treatment has to be repeated every four to six months.

Lazy girl's sweat relief

1. To avoid embarrassing sweat patches, especially around your groin, armpit and back, try the following:
2. Avoid wearing light-coloured clothes if you know you're prone to sweat. Also make sure your clothes are made of cotton, as this absorbs sweat, and are relatively loose as opposed to skin-tight Lycra, which traps sweat and makes it literally run down your body in rivulets.
3. Use a strong antiperspirant, not a deodorant, as the latter is basically just a perfume spray, whereas an antiperspirant will slow down your perspiration.
4. Shave your armpits, as hair can make BO worse because it traps bacteria.
5. Finally, use an antibacterial soap to zap bacteria and help you avoid BO.

Varicose veins

Although varicose veins in the legs grow progressively worse with age, they can appear as early as in your twenties. They occur because veins in the lower body are lined with valves that help blood return to the heart. The superficial veins running just beneath the skin take back 10 per cent of blood and the deep veins take the remaining 90 per cent. For the blood to return against the flow of gravity there are one-way valves positioned along the walls of the vein. When these walls become slack, the valves don't shut properly and blood flows backwards and pools in the veins. The good news is varicose veins have no symptoms, apart from bulging veins, though some sufferers do have aches in the affected areas.

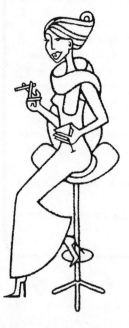

To get rid of bulgy veins, a simple and quick operation is performed. This can be done if the vein is causing discomfort or appears unflattering. For milder cases wearing support tights is recommended, as this can relieve the ache and may improve the appearance by flattening the veins.

To prevent it in the first place:

- Do not sit or stand for a long time, as this puts undue strain on your leg veins.
- Keep your weight down, as weight puts pressure on vein walls.
- Do regular exercise, as this promotes good circulation in the legs.
- Stop smoking, as smoking interferes with blood flow.

Thread veins and spider veins

More or less everyone gets thread veins as they get older. Though some people are naturally more prone to them, as they're hereditary (so blame your mum). They are most commonly found in women – and around one in five women in their twenties have them running around the thigh and leg area. In most cases no one else will ever notice them but you. However, if they bug you or you can't bear showing your legs, there are things you can do to improve the skin:

Sclerotherapy is a non-surgical treatment that was developed in the 1920s to get rid of what are known as thread or spider veins. The technique is performed with a micro-needle and a solution of either some kind of saline or something known as a sclerosant. This is injected into the vein to turn it white and make the vein collapse and disappear.

A typical treatment lasts 30 minutes and is what's known as a lunchtime procedure, meaning you can have it done and go straight back to work. Though be wary of going to a step class or for a run, as it's recommended that you wait at least 24 hours before taking strenuous exercise. Also bear in mind that you'll need three to four treatments for the best results and may have to wear some sturdy support stockings during the next day to help prevent bruising.

For smaller veins a new technique known as pulsed dye laser is used. Again, this is a lunchtime treatment during which a laser is pointed at your veins and a light beam is directed into the area causing the vessel walls to seal up, thereby stopping blood flowing into the small thread-like veins. It feels kind of tingly and doesn't hurt, but you do have to avoid the sun after treatment.

More body hair

Good old body hair; if you're not blitzing in the name of beauty from your face, underarms and legs, you have to defuzz it from other inexplicable places. The good news is, unless you have hair growing on your palms or the soles of your feet, you are perfectly normal. And unless the hair is sprouting in large thatch-like patches, you can relax and defuzz (if it *is* sprouting see your doctor: you could have a slight hormonal imbalance).

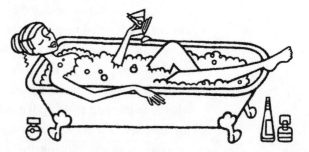

Nipple hair: it's very common to have the odd sparse hair sprout around the areola, and this can quite safely be plucked or trimmed and it won't grow back stronger or heavier. If you find fine baby hair, leave it where it is; no one will ever notice it but you.

tip

Never shave body hair along your belly line unless you want to sprout a stubbly shadow from your navel to your private bits.

Hair in strange places

Belly button line: stomach hairs are very common and usually lie in a line from your belly button to your groin. If you hate the look of it, wax it away. This is the most efficient way to avoid the stubble effect and get a smooth finish. Always apply wax in the direction of hair growth and hold the skin taut as you pull back in the opposite direction. Afterwards soothe your skin with aloe vera so you don't replace the hair with a red line.

Above your bottom: ever felt that Fuzzyfelt patch above your bottom and at the base of your spine? If it's more fuzzy than soft you can defuzz here as well. Again, try a wax job. Ask a friend to help or go for a depilatory cream; although you may have to twist like a contortionist for it to work well.

Under your thighs: lots of women have downy hair here. It's easy to get rid of via shaving creams or waxing; the question is – is it worth it?

Body hair that keeps coming back

Well, body hair *does* keep coming back because that's its job. If you're sick of it, consider laser treatments. They work by shooting a beam of light towards the desired area, which in turn destroys the hair follicle. It will take a few sessions to zap the hair for good or at least retard its growth, but some girls say it's worth it. Bear in mind, though, that follicles do get replaced so it's not permanent in a forever sense. To thin hair out, there is a variety of creams that stunt hair growth. If used regularly they can eventually make even the hairiest beastette need her shaver less frequently. Look for hair-inhibiting creams. These help reduce the growth of hair, and though they take time to work, they eventually do the job effectively.

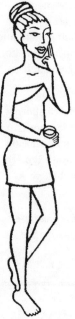

Face blips

Dark circles under the eyes

The giveaway sign that you're probably the number-one party girl is dark circles under the eyes. The problem is the skin underneath your eyes is so thin that the blood vessels below show up, especially when you're tired or hungover.

You can boost the strength of this skin by: using creams that contain antioxidants, such as vitamin C and soya; better still you can do the lie-back-and-rest technique that involves camomile and cucumber patches over your eyes (use cucumber slices or cotton-wool pads soaked in cold camomile tea). These firm up the eye area and constrict the blood vessels so they become less noticeable. Then get some more sleep – eight hours a night for a week works a treat.

Morning breath

Whether or not this is nature's cruel way of making morning sex unappealing, the truth is only a few of us are immune to bad breath when we wake up, usually the result of the lack of saliva, snoring and drooling unappealingly on our pillows. Apart from alcohol, smoking, garlic and a midnight kebab, rancid halitosis is caused by a build-up of bacteria that naturally occurs overnight while you're sleeping. If you breathe through your mouth while you sleep you don't generate enough saliva to wash away germs in the mouth – something that happens naturally by day. This helps cultivate a bacterial build-up, usually at the back of the tongue, which is the cause of the vile vapours. Possible solutions include scrubbing your tongue as you clean your teeth and using a mouthwash.

If your rancid breath lasts all day, then you could have a problem with tooth decay and gum disease. This is the number-one cause of bad breath and is easily solved by a trip to your dentist, the regular use of dental floss and drinking a good amount of water a day.

tip

If all else fails in your quest for fresh breath, try buying a tongue scraper (weird metal arch). Pull this along your tongue to clear the tongue. Revolting but it works.

Scars from zits

It's not uncommon for a zit to leave an unsightly blemish in its place. It's usually the result of much concealer dabbing and scraping 'accidentally on purpose' with your nails. On certain skin types – black and Asian in particular – the scarring looks worse because the skin's pigmentation doesn't match up and so you seem to be left with a permanent reminder of what was once there. To prevent post-pimple problems, start by avoiding the obvious: don't pick! To pop a zit successfully, do it using cotton wool and/or

Spot cover-up

To get a flawless face is harder than just slapping on some concealer. Do it wrongly and all you're doing is changing a red bulbous spot into a brown bulbous spot. To conceal effectively:

1. Buy a concealer that exactly matches your skin – never go paler, as it simply highlights your problem area.
2. Don't rub it in or wipe it across your face, but pat it into your blemish. With spots, paint over with a fine brush.
3. Apply after foundation so you don't wipe it off when you're rubbing in your make-up.
4. To mask big scars and spots, use an opaque concealer and apply with a foundation sponge (bought at any chemist).

tissues instead of nails and pull away rather than squeeze inwards. Better still, dry out the spot using a benzoyl peroxide-based product. If the red marks persist and the skin looks flaky, use a hydrocortisone cream every day for a week. This will soothe the skin and help get rid of the mark, and remember to use a sunscreen over the red area if you're going out into the sun, as the sun will just discolour it further.

tip

If the dark circles under your eye won't go away no matter how much sleep you get, see your GP it could be a sign of bad circulation or another underlying problem.

Cold sores

Most people develop immunity to cold sores as kids, but for some unknown reason a third of the population never acquires immunity, meaning cold-sore outbreaks. If you're prone to open sores on your lips, it's worth knowing that you aren't catching a new virus each time but you are reactivating an old virus, which lies dormant in the facial nerves until it's triggered again. Cold-sore triggers are: sunlight, stress, colds and illnesses. If you're adept at noticing your body's warnings you may feel a slight tingling sensation 24 hours before a blister appears; if so slap on the cold-sore treatment now – available over the counter in pharmacies.

If you haven't been able to zap it immediately, consider preventative steps:

1. Always put sunscreen on your lips, as the UV rays in sunlight trigger the virus.

2. Ask your doctor for a prescription drug or buy an over-the-counter product.

3. Avoid picking at it or else you'll end up with a secondary infection.

4. To disguise a cold sore, never apply powder, as it will make the sore look dry and emphasise it. However, do use a lip balm to keep it moist (but don't share it). A normal one will do or use an antibiotic ointment.

Drooping cheeks

Cheeks that droop, are, again, a by-product of ageing, hereditary factors and a life lived on the edge of healthiness. The good news is you can help stop your cheeks reaching your chin, and dragging your upper face down with them, by boosting facial firmness. The answer here is simple: do some exercise. The elasticity of skin (the snapback theory: pull your skin out and see if it snaps back or takes a leisurely stroll back) amongst women who work out three days a week is not only better than that of non-exercisers but also near on age-defying. This is because skin is an organ, and, like other organs, it needs a healthy flow of oxygen and exercise to firm it up. Think of your face like your backside: work it hard and it will remain pert and upright.

Hair blips

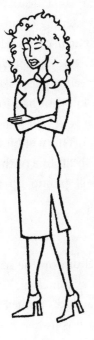

Frizzy hair

Unless you're born with natural frizz (and many people are), frizzy hair is usually the result of bad hair management. Roughly translated this means you have blitzed it with a hairdryer, blasted it in the sun or loaded it with chemicals from colourants and products. Little wonder then that your hair is now going crazy.

The good news is that even the fiercest hairbear can be tamed with a variety of hair products. First up are conditioners and balms that contain panthenol, or silicone-based products to coat the cuticle and help it to lie flat. Simply rub it through wet or dry hair and your hair will be frizz-free. This technique works effectively, but use too much product or allow a build-up of the balm – by not shampooing properly – and you'll have the opposite problem of lank hair.

Other conditioners, which do the same but with a lighter hand, include those with shea butter and seed oils; these again seal the cuticles, erasing frizz and leaving you with either Pre-Raphaelite curls or hair straighter than a piece of string. As for blow-drying, help yourself by pointing your hairdryer downwards as it blows, so the hair lies flat, and NEVER EVER hold the dryer against the hair unless you want your hair to go into a frizz frenzy.

Limp hair

When hair goes flat, lank and as limp as a dead fish, products are to blame. Too much straightening serum or heavy use of conditioner will pull your hair down. Help yourself by either switching to a light one or applying conditioner to only your ends. If you're feeling particularly brave, skip it altogether – it really won't kill your hair for a couple of days to go without. Then wash your hair as normal and blow-dry the roots with cold air. This will lift the hair and give you that extra lift as well. To lift fine or thinning hair, consider a colour, which will plump up the cuticles and improve the condition.

Oily hair

This occurs when there is too much sebum on the scalp and it ends up layering the hair shaft and making your head feel dirty, as the oil attracts dirt that sticks to the hair shaft. The best way to avoid this is to wash your hair every day. Contrary to popular myth this does not encourage your hair to produce more oil. An every-day shampoo should be used if you have an oily scalp, and/or if you exercise every day and if you have very fine hair.

Look at the ingredients on your shampoo and make sure you avoid panthenol and silicone products, which just make the hair look and feel more oily.

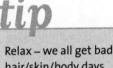

Dry hair

When you hair is dying for a drink, dry hair is the sign. To hydrate, just feed it moisture. This means less shampoo, which can dry hair out, and more conditioner, preferably one that you can leave in. Also watch how you dry your hair and think about sun protection. Nine times out of ten, dry hair is the result of environmental hazards, such as the sun's rays. Use a hair sunscreen or a hat, and deep-condition once a week. Overall, practise gentleness when styling. Do not brush hair when it's wet: it causes hair to break. Use a detangler if you are combing wet, curly hair, let hair dry naturally for five to ten minutes before styling and, finally, get a trim every six weeks.

Thinning hair

Hair loss is caused by a variety of factors: ageing, stress, bad diet, illness and allergies to hair products. However, in most cases it's the result of iron and protein deficiencies, which means you need to eat a healthier diet and forgo habits such as smoking and too much drinking if you want lush hair. If you've already gone down this path, it's worth considering a visit to your doctor, as the cause could be hormonal and therefore easily corrected with medication. There are also shampoos on the market, which can help: look for a product called Regaine, which has to be applied daily. It's not instantaneous so give it six months if you decide to go down that route.

Hand and nail blips

Ridged nails

The nail plate is made up of three layers, and when you accidentally bash your nails and trap them in car doors you'll find yourself with uneven waves across them. In most cases ridged nails are actually hereditary, and the best way to improve the look of the nail is to keep your nails short and buff down the ridges with a nail buffer. This looks like a nail file but has three different surfaces. You buff with each of them to create a smooth nail plate, but only do this twice a month or you'll damage the nail.

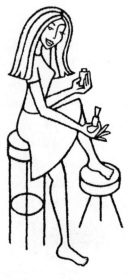

White spots

There are a multitude of reasons for the appearance of white spots, including, say some experts, a lack of calcium and zinc. However, in most cases bruising the nail plate is to blame. Usually, you can leave the marked nail to grow itself out. If you're plagued with them, go down the preventative route and be aware of how you treat your hands. Nasty bangs and drumming of nails can damage the nail plate and cause the very spots you're trying to rid yourself of.

Discoloured nails

Use too many dark nail polishes and/or smoke and you're asking for yellowing nails. The easy solution is to either remove your nail polish every night and/or use a base coat to protect the nails from discoloration. If it's too late for that, wipe over them with lemon juice and then buff (see Ridged Nails, above), but after buffing always ensure you use a protection layer (base or top coat) before applying new colour.

Lifestyle blips

Hangover looks

Do any of the following sound familiar?

- Greasy, lank hair.
- Greyish, sallow skin.
- A papery texture to the surface of your skin.
- Red eyes.
- Dry mouth.
- Bad breath.
- Aching limbs.

If so, you're currently experiencing the beauty effects of a hangover. While we've all been there, it might help to know why you look this way. Firstly, the acid in the alcohol is irritating your stomach which is why your skin is rebelling and looking vile. Secondly, dry mouth and papery skin occurs because the alcohol in your body has acted like a diuretic and made you pee too much.

To avoid looking like an ageing film star ...

... boost your looks by:

- Plastering on the moisturiser. Your skin is crying out for a drink, so apply lashings to your face and balm to your lips.
- Look after your eyes. Zap dark circles and red eyes with slices of cucumber placed over the eyes and eye drops to refresh and hydrate them.
- Avoid a face full of make-up. Apart from the fact you'll look scary, your make-up is likely to be a shade too dark, as blood is circulated away from the skin to help your body cope with detoxifying. If you have to wear something, avoid powders – they will just make your skin look drier, and go for the simple lip-gloss-and-sunglasses look.
- Tie your hair up. Alcohol excretes through your pores so hair may feel greasy and lank. Tie it up or pull it back to avoid having to feel it all day.
- Eat some vegetables and fruit. Antioxidants are particularly apt at fighting off alcohol damage and protecting your liver. They also strengthen the resilience of your skin. Found in green leafy vegetables and fruit. Aim to get ample amounts of vitamins A, C and E in the days before a big night out.
- Drink more water. This will help rid your body of the toxin acetaldehyde, which is released by the liver when alcohol is broken down. It is this toxin that causes your dehydrated look.

Travel tips — how to fly and still look gorgeous

Only the very few can get off a plane and look stunning after a long flight. If you don't have a big hat and a pair of sunglasses handy, you need to inject a serious beauty routine into your flying technique. The problem is in-flight cabin humidity. This means in-flight dehydration is one of the most serious hazards of flying for your skin, hair and energy levels. While you can't avoid the fact your body will become dehydrated, the following can help you to stay hydrated:

- Opt for a 250 ml (8 fl oz) glass of water every hour. Alcohol and coffee also have a diuretic effect so make sure you have a bottle of water with you (so you don't have to rely on the drinks trolley).
- Apply almond oil or Vaseline to the inside of your nostrils to help lubricate the nasal membranes. This will stop them from drying out.
- For dry, sore eyes, dampen a piece of muslin or a face cloth and regularly place it over your skin to keep it cool and moist.

To avoid the sallow skin and limp hair of air travel and jet lag:

- Exercise before you go on a long flight, as it's beneficial to your body. It improves the body's circulation, increases the body's metabolic rate and boosts energy levels; all of these things will help to combat fatigue.

- On arrival at your destination, aim to keep your body going, especially if you've gained time, i.e. you're travelling to a place where it's still day. A long walk in the sunshine or even a swim will keep your energy levels constant, which is good news for your holiday looks.

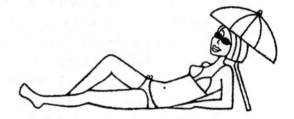

20 ways
to recover and repair

1 Blitz your scaly bits
Sandpaper feet and scabby knees and elbows can destroy the look of the best beauty goddess. To soothe and soften, rub Vaseline into the dry areas before getting into a bath. Afterwards your skin will be soft and smooth.

2 Don't get stressed
Tension can make you break out, lose skin moisture, appear sallow and even age faster, as it causes blood vessels to contract and impairs the skin's ability to stay moist.

3 Take ten minutes' sofa time a day for your skin
Yup, you heard that right – lie on the sofa. When you're worked up and stressed out you'll break out. This is because stress stimulates the sebaceous glands, which in turn leads to spots. (This is usually why you also get spots before a hot date and around your period.)

4 Over-plucked brows
A serious contender for number-one beauty disaster. If you've over-plucked your eyebrows, don't be tempted to equal them up so they look the same. Instead grin and bear it. Eyebrows don't take long to grow back. In the meantime use Vaseline to keep your brows in place and, if they look very bare, fill in the gaps lightly with a pencil the shade of your brow.

5 Brighten hangover eyes
Easily achieved with zero effort. Simply use a pale eyeshadow on the lower inner corners of your eyes, if you have dark eyes. For lighter eyes use a non-black mascara on your lashes. It's much softer on the eyes and brings out your eye colour.

6 Avoid lipstick on your teeth
Horrible beauty disaster, but easy to avoid. Simply apply your lipstick and then put your forefinger in your mouth. Wrap your inner lips around it, and drag your finger out. It will remove the colour from only the inside of your lips.

7 Close your pores

Hot weather can open even the smallest pores and make you look like 13 years old again (but not in a good way). To stop the enlarged look, after you wash your face run an ice cube over it to constrict the pores, then use an oil-controlling product beneath your moisturiser and/or sunscreen.

8 Pass the daylight test

That mirror in your bedroom may make you look gorgeous, but does your make-up pass the daylight test, i.e. how natural is that foundation you're applying so liberally. Help yourself by putting make-up on in natural light, not a bright mirror light.

9 Salvage a make-up disaster

You've applied your make-up too heavily and have no time to start again. Easy, get some tissues and gently press against your skin to blot off excess lip-stick, eyeshadow and foundation. If that doesn't do the trick, dampen a muslin cloth and press again.

10 Get your brows right

Eyebrows should start from the outer edge of your nose. Place your fore-finger at your nostril in a straight line to find the exact point. Over this area screams 'horror film', too far the other way screams 'disaster'.

11 Condition your hair before flying

Tie hair back and slick with leave-in conditioner to protect it from dry aeroplane air. Wash it off as soon as you hit your destination and you'll have super-lush hair.

12 To smooth out smudged nails

Dip your finger in nail-polish remover very quickly. The colour will then even out on its own.

13 Untanned spaces on your tanned body

Get rid of telltale bikini-strap marks by using self-tan on the tanned bits. Even better, apply self-tan and then brush on a bronzing powder to really keep the white bits covered up.

14 Soothe prickly heat

Get rid of the red rash that appears in the sun (usually on the torso, arms, legs and under the bra straps) by using a cotton-wool ball soaked in cold tea and then replenish your body's water supply so that you rehydrate the skin from inside.

15 Zapping the zits on your bottom

Embarrassing but very real. Use a skin exfoliator on your derrière. Try one that you can apply before you get into the bath that also applies moisture to the area. Good ones include the creams that contain seeds. You can also use a pumice stone.

16 Keep teeth white

By drinking juices and colas through a straw. The straw delivers the liquid directly to the back of your throat, giving the acid and sugar in your drinks less time to erode your pearly whites.

17 Hone your hand care

Shorten your soaks in the bath and always wear Marigolds when you wash up. Nails become weak and soft when immersed in water for too long. If you're going for a long soak, read a book to keep your hands out of the water.

18 File nails, don't cut

Filing causes less stress to the nail, plus gives you a better shape so you can have sexy-looking talons.

19 Protect your nails

If you're going to do some gardening or DIY, protect your nails from dirt and grime by scraping them over a bar of soap first. This will act as a barrier to nasties.

20 Avoid red shaving bumps

Especially on your legs and along the bikini line, by exfoliating with a coarse face cloth or exfoliator before you shave. Remember to apply, wash off and then use shaving foam before shaving. Soothe the area afterwards with aloe vera and keep exfoliating for the following two days.

chapter 7
Pampering

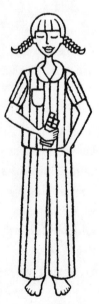

Good beauty is not just about make-up techniques, beauty cover-ups and looking gorgeous. It's also about feeling gorgeous, which means beauty equals pampering yourself. If the thought of soaking in a hot bath infused with petals, rubbing expensive lotions into your skin and wafting about smelling of roses does it for you, then you know what I am talking about. However, if you feel stressed, tired, depressed and fed up, it's unlikely you've got to grips with the art of spoiling yourself just for the sake of it. Which is why, even if you do nothing else in the name of beauty, it pays to pamper. Tempted to give it a go? Well, this is the chapter for you.

What's what with spas

Spas, health farms, retreats, alternative-therapy centres – they're not only everywhere but also they cater for every type of person. From the stressed-out celeb who gets her kicks spending zillions a night to the knackered party girl who needs a break that doesn't involve alcohol and another late night.

A spa is basically the lazy girl's beauty haven; a place where you can lounge around in a bathrobe all day, intermittently soaking yourself in the Jacuzzi and then popping along for the odd treatment. It's the beauty equivalent of a top-notch gym, complete with experts on hand to do everything from pummel you into relaxation, de-stress your face, cleanse your pores, irrigate your digestion, paint your toenails, pluck your brows and smooth out your wrinkles. Of course, spas aren't for everyone, especially if you don't have a pot full of money to give away. However, if you do manage to raid your piggy bank, here are the treatments to look out for – all are also available at day salons:

The massage therapies

Massage can help a variety of problems suffered by the tired, stressed and aching body. Getting to know which ones help which problem will make your decision at the spa easier.

Thai massage

What is it? This technique is over 1,000 years old and is related to acupuncture, Hatha yoga and Ayurvedic medicine. Unlike other forms of massage, Thai therapy uses a mixture of acupressure, body rocking and deep, assisted yoga-like stretches, to open the whole body. The focus is on the musculo-skeletal system – the bones, joints, muscles and connective tissue – and the aim is to release tension in all these areas so you can feel healthier all round. The massage takes about one hour and is carried out on the floor; you can remain clothed or unclothed. Apart from helping you to relax, Thai massage can also help to aid sleep, decrease stress and boost energy.

Health benefits: excellent for skin radiance, relieving headaches, neck and shoulder aches, and insomnia.

Sports massage

What is it? A deep body massage (performed directly on to the skin) designed to prevent sports injuries and enhance an athlete's performance. Sports massage works on the premise that lactic and carbonic acids build up in the muscle tissue during exercise causing pain and fatigue. They need to be removed so that the body can work effectively. This technique involves a variety of deep kneading, stroking, shaking and manipulation movements designed to soften muscles and promote flexibility around the joints. Pressure is applied with elbows, hands and the body weight of the practitioner.

Health benefits: the massage softens muscle fibres, improves flexibility and boosts energy, leaving you feeling and looking fantastic.

tip

If you're booking into a spa check what your room fee includes as many spas ask for extra money for treatments.

The spa checklist

Before trusting your beauty and body to someone, check out the following:

1. Ensure the therapist always asks questions about your health before a treatment. Make sure you mention any illnesses and injuries and whether you are pregnant or taking medication prior to treatment (especially if the treatment is to do with heating the body or rubbing something into the skin).
2. Ask if she is fully insured to practise and has been trained (her certificates should be on display). If she is not, do not let her near you.
3. Make sure she is a member of a professional organisation, and check her membership with the organisation.
4. Read up on the treatment before going along so you know what to expect.
5. Ask if there is anything you shouldn't do before a treatment; for example, if you are having your skin waxed, you should avoid overheating your skin in a sauna or in an exercise class.

myth

Massage is just some person rubbing your body until you fall asleep. Untrue. While there are namby-pamby massages that do the above, the majority of therapeutic massages literally pummel the body into shape. This means falling asleep will be the last thing on your mind. Read descriptions carefully before plonking your naked body down on a bed.

Shiatsu

What is it? Shiatsu means 'finger pressure' and is a non-invasive form of massage that originates from Japan. Based on the principle that the body's energy flows through lines – or meridians – in the body, the aim of Shiatsu is to apply pressure to these lines to boost your energy and benefit your general health. The massage is performed on the floor and you remain fully clothed throughout.

Health benefits: it's especially good for regulating the autonomic nervous system, which governs the heart, breathing and blood pressure, giving you an amazing radiant glow.

Indian champissage head massage

What is it? Indian head champissage is based on the 1,000-year-old Ayurvedic healing system, though the form practised now also incorporates a massage of the neck, shoulders and arms as well as the head. The massage is performed through light clothing, in a seated position and without the use of any oils, and involves the kneading and rubbing of the shoulder, head and neck muscles and the massaging of the scalp and hair follicles.

Health benefits: the aim is to release toxins and built-up stress in the body's muscles. It will rejuvenate your looks instantaneously.

What's what with aromatherapy oils

- To wake you up – grapefruit.
- To make you sleepy – lavender.
- To give you energy – lemon.
- To make you feel nurtured – rose.
- To clear your mind – eucalyptus.
- To get rid of mosquitoes – citronella.

NB: if you are going to apply the oil to your skin, always mix it first with a base oil such as almond oil.

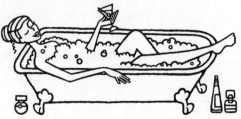

The fake tanners

Avoid skin cancer and still look fab by trying out a fake tan treatment. These days most are designed to fade into something more natural so don't freak at the initial effects.

St Tropez tan

The process begins with being scrubbed down with an exfoliator so your skin is baby-soft for the application process. Next step is the slapping on of the sludgy stuff, which is basically plastered on head to toe. Wear a thong for maximum effect and expect to resemble a mud monster for the next hour. Leave the stuff on all night (probably best not to have white sheets) and then shower off in the morning, and you should be left with an even, brown tan. If it's applied properly it should last for seven to ten days.

Fake bake

Again, it starts with an exfoliation and then a reddish-brown gloop is applied to your body. To seal in the colour, you are then spritzed with an oil-based spray. The colour should then develop around six hours later and should look natural rather than orange. The effects last for around a week.

Su-do airbrush tan

The human equivalent of getting your car resprayed. It involves standing in various positions for half an hour while you're sprayed with a tan. Again the colour takes about five hours to develop and lasts around ten days.

The tan rules — how to make your fake tan last

1. Don't shower or swim until 12 hours after a treatment.
2. If you're going to apply it yourself make sure you cover all areas.
3. Wear dark clothing unless you want tidemarks on your clothes.
4. If you're doing it for a special occasion, do it a few days before the event, to get a more natural look.
5. Patch-test an area of your body for allergies and effect before you plaster your whole body.

tip

The best time to go to a Spa is during the week in an off peak season such as February as this is when you can find the best deals.

The exercise therapies

Yoga and Pilates are gentle forms of exercise that are good for building muscle strength and toning the body. There are several forms of yoga, which range from very gentle stretching to highly active movements. Both yoga and Pilates should be considered as part of a regular exercise programme, not just when you visit a spa, but you may want to sample them there to see which ones appeal to you.

myth

Yoga and Pilates are only for the very fit and agile. Untrue. The joy of these exercises is that they are adaptable, which is why they are excellent for pregnant women, people who have been injured, the unfit and those who are recovering from an operation. Always ensure you speak to a teacher before class, so they can tailor the exercises to your needs.

Astanga yoga

Often described as power yoga, Astanga is the most physically demanding form of yoga. It's also the most cardiovascular, because it's based around a dynamic continuous flow of movements and postures and is not about standing still in an incense-filled room. It also has the most noticeable results. Many of the postures are extremely difficult and take time and practice to master correctly.

Sivananda and Jivamukti yoga

These two forms of yoga have greater spiritual emphasis than other types of yoga and therefore attract the deeper thinkers of the yoga pack. The emphasis is mainly on meditation and clearing the mind of rubbish. However, as

Sivananda and Jivamukti are also both based on a very traditional form of Hatha yoga (see below), both also couple very athletic moves with the incense-scented ritual. Jivamukti in particular focuses on breathing as a way to stretch out the body.

Hatha yoga

The most accessible type of yoga and the one you're most likely to find at a local evening class is Hatha yoga. The word derives from 'ha' meaning 'sun' and 'tha' meaning 'moon', and together they mean 'union'. This is a term used to describe a central form of yoga that combines lots of different types of positions.

Iyengar yoga

A slow and precise form of yoga, Iyengar may look easy and simple to the beginner but it is tightly controlled, consisting of 12 movements, which need to be mastered and held (i.e. no wobbling on the spot). Props, such as ballet barres and walls, are often used to help people maintain and find their balance. Once mastered, Iyengar yoga is said to give you 'muscles of steel', fantastic alignment, good posture and a meditative state of mind.

Kundalini yoga

In this yoga, breath work and relaxation is reached through a series of postures and chanting. Kundalini yoga is said to be fantastic for prenatal mums. It's also a way to turn back the clock and erase the years, as the guru behind this form of yoga, Gurmukh Kaur Khalsa, is 60 but looks as if she is in her late thirties. 'Do Kundalini,' she advocates, 'and you never have to grow old.' Said to be the best for good karma and spiritualism.

Bikram yoga

The main principle of Bikram yoga is that heat will help aid movement, flexibility and breathing. For this reason classes take place in rooms heated to around 38 degrees Celsius (100 degrees Fahrenheit). The aim is also to help the body sweat out toxins; meaning the classes are very smelly indeed.

Pilates

A sister form of exercise to yoga that aims to lengthen and strengthen the body, Pilates is good for improving posture and back injuries and is fantastic for toning. It can be done as a mat class, which incorporates floor-based Pilates exercises (up to 500 of them) or as a resistance class with machines. The basis of Pilates is to create a strong 'core', or abdominal muscles, which not only helps support the spine but also aligns the body. To get the best out of a class it's essential to get a teacher who has practised Pilates for years and has been trained for at least two years (for international teachers go to UK websites in resources).

Osteopathy

This is a treatment that is based on the body's structure (the skeleton, muscles and connective tissue). Osteopaths use their hands to treat the body, manipulating soft tissue and mobilising joints. It's excellent for the back, repetitive strain injury (RSI), joint pain and sports injuries. On the beauty side, it will literally make you stand tall and give you amazing posture.

The facials

There are hundreds of different types of facials on offer at spas and salons, and all work on the basis that they cleanse, moisturise and help rejuvenate skin. To pick the one that's right for you will depend on cost, your skin type and the kind of treatment you're looking for. To help you make up your mind, consider the following:

1. If you have broken, ultra-sensitive skin and/or are allergic to many skin creams and cleansers, avoid facials, no matter what the therapist says. The chances are she will aggravate your skin condition without realising it.
2. Don't let therapists sell you an entire new range of skincare, especially if the products you've been using have been working fine. They may believe in the products, but no one range of

skincare is better than another. Also, to be brutally honest, they make commission on sales. If they are adamant the products are good for you, ask for samples to try out at home first.

3. Make sure you know all the details of the facial before you begin. Some involve face masks and eye masks and can be claustrophobic if you're not used to them. Also, some – the Cathiodermie in particular – involve facial rollers that conduct a minute electrical current, which can look alarming if you haven't been forewarned.

4. Be realistic about what a facial can do. In most cases it will be a thorough cleansing/moisturising, skin-stimulating treatment, but it doesn't have the power to get rid of spots or facial lines.

5. Finally, if at any time during a facial your skin begins to sting or itch, don't just assume it's the facial, tell the therapist right away, as it could be an allergic reaction.

The lazy girl's DIY facial

The essentials: a large kitchen bowl, towel, muslin cloth (buy from baby shops), oats, almond oil, avocado, banana, cucumber slices and rose oil.

Step one: fill the bowl with hot water (if you use boiling water add cold to the mix). Lean over the bowl and place a towel over your head and bowl, so you have trapped the steam and are steaming your face (if the steam is too hot to bear, add cold water).

Step two: when the water cools down, dip the muslin cloth into the water, wring out and place the cloth over your face. Breathe in and out for five counts. Repeat three times.

Step three: mix the oats with some almond oil and use as an exfoliating scrub. Use cold water to wash off.

Step four: mash up the avocado and banana, and use as a face mask (you may need to use some oil to help it bond). Place two cucumber slices over your eyes and lie down for ten minutes.

Step five: rinse your face with warm water and pat dry.

Step six: now add three drops of rose oil into six drops of almond oil and smooth on as a moisturiser (if it's too oily, use a tissue to soak up the excess).

tip

Lazy girl number one pampering tip: Turn off phone, lie on sofa in PJs and eat chocolate at least once every month.

The body therapies

Ayurvedic medicine

Meaning 'the science of life', Ayurveda is a holistic method of treating illness. Each patient is assessed via a process that analyses their constitution and lifestyle rather than just focusing on their symptoms. Treatment is given through dietary advice, supplements, massage and meditation.

Good for: allergies, skin complaints, and headaches.

LaStone therapy

Dating back to 2,000 BC, LaStone therapy is a healing treatment, which uses heated stones (volcanic black basalt) or cooled stones (white marble) to relax and soothe the body. The modern version was developed in Arizona and the idea is for the stones to relieve tense and tired muscles. The theory being the heat from the stones permeates through the muscle, soothing tensions and strains. The stones are then soaked in oil and stroked over the body to increase circulation. It has been found that one stroke of a stone is worth 13 by hand and, therefore, the treatment is much more intense and effective than other relaxing therapies.

Good for: very stressed types who need to let go.

Acupuncture

The practice of acupuncture involves placing sterilised fine needles into the skin, along the body's energy pathways – meridians – in order to clear problems/illnesses. In beauty spas it's used mainly for relaxation.

Good for: PMS, fatigue, skin conditions.

Aromatherapy

This therapy involves the application of various plant essential oils – about 400 of them in total – which, when mixed with a base oil and applied to the skin, help cause changes within the body's enzymes. Do not try if you are pregnant.

Good for: fatigue, stress and PMS.

Reflexology

This is the practice of applying pressure to points on the feet and hands (which correspond to various areas of the body) to stimulate the body and induce relaxation as well as heal.

Good for: tiredness, stress and long-term well-being.

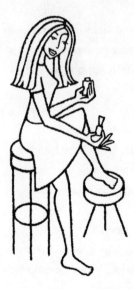

20 ways to create the spa effect on the cheap

1 Stock up on samples
Ask make-up counters to let you try products before you buy them and then have a beauty night to see what works and what doesn't.

2 Go local
For a sauna and steam room seek out your local swimming pool where there is always at least one, if not both of the above.

3 Find a student masseur
For a massage, find a local training school where students are supervised and offer a massage at a discounted rate.

4 Raid the kitchen
For the spa feeling, have one at home. Use rock salt to exfoliate, an avocado face mask to hydrate and honey to cleanse.

5 Invest in a beauty therapist for the night
Call a local beautician and ask her if she'd give you a discount rate for you and some friends if you arrange a beauty party where all the guests pay her for treatments.

6 Have a beauty pot-luck night
Everyone pays five pounds so you can buy an array of beauty products, and then everyone tries them out round at your house. Think pedicures, manicures, face masks.

7 Go mid-week to a spa
Nearly every health farm gives discounted rates for Sunday through to Thursday when they are least busy. This is a good time to try one out on the cheap.

8 Try treatments abroad
Spa treatments are usually a lot cheaper when you're on holiday, especially if you book a local speciality.

9 Think about going for a day

Many spas have day passes, where you can get all of the above for half the price.

10 Buy cheaper versions of the posh products

They work just as well and at half the price.

11 Better still make your own spa products

For a face pack, go for mashed banana and honey. For a body scrub, use porridge oats, massage oil and a ripe avocado. To come out smelling sweetly, place a herbal tea bag under the bath tap to infuse your place with herbal smells.

12 Have a head-to-toe day

Spend the whole day smoothing, cleansing and moisturising your body. Start in the morning with your hair, and move down each part of your body as the day progresses, making sure to leave time to simply lounge around in your bathrobe watching videos.

13 Join a gym

You may never hit the treadmill, but you can use the pool, the sauna, and the steam room and check out the beauty area all at a lower fee than a normal spa.

14 Buy a book on massage

The joy of massage is anyone can learn to do it. Study up on a massage manual and then swap treatments with friends.

15 Give yourself a foot rub

Don't underestimate the power of rubbing your feet. To get the rub right, use some peppermint or tea tree oil and massage your feet by rubbing along the inner arch, on to the ball of the foot and along the toes. When you're done, massage on the moisturiser and put on some cotton socks. By morning you'll have perfect feet.

16 Go without make-up for the whole weekend

. . . and styling products and perfume, and just let your body breathe for the day. You may have to stay hidden in your back garden but it will be worth it by Monday morning.

17 Get eight whole hours of sleep a night

For one entire weekend – that's Friday night to Monday morning – go to bed and sleep for eight hours each night. By Monday you'll look as if you've been relaxing at a Caribbean spa for the weekend.

18 Use lavender oil

Want to feel truly relaxed and laid back? Then rub on some lavender oil (mix it with a base oil first). It promotes relaxation and feelings of well-being and will help you to sleep easy.

19 Laugh more

It will give your facial muscles a workout, make you look radiant, improve your skin tone and generally make you more fanciable to the opposite sex.

20 Stop worrying about your looks

Rich advice from a beauty book, I know, but the truth is fixating on your looks is the number-one beauty killer. The key to beauty is simple: cleanse, moisturise, eat well, take some exercise, drink plenty of water, wear sunscreen, get some sleep and then forget about the beauty stuff and get on with your life!

chapter 8

How to be extremely knowledgeable about beauty (without trying)

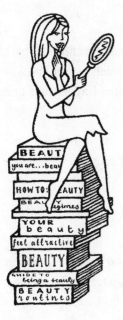

Too lazy to focus on the relevant chapters? Well then, this section's for you: a simple A–Z of all the beauty jargon with lazy-girl translations.

Acupuncture

Technical version: acupuncture involves placing sterilised fine needles into the skin, along the body's energy pathways – meridians – in order to help with problems/ illnesses. Used more as a relaxant in the beauty stakes.

Lazy girl's version: needles plunged into your skin in the name of relaxation.

AHAs

Technical version: also known as alpha hydroxy acids. These acids work by speeding up cell renewal and exfoliating the top layer of skin.

Lazy girl's version: fruit acids that dissolve the top layer of skin to make your face look smoother and brighter.

Alexander technique

Technical version: a postural realignment technique that's less effort than yoga or Pilates. It teaches you the key beauty technique: good posture in standing, sitting and getting up.

Lazy girl's version: how to appear 10 cm (4 in) taller than you are, and get out of a car without showing your knickers.

Antioxidants

Technical version: antioxidants, found in foods, creams and now certain drinks, work by mopping up the damage free radicals (see below) do to your body. Keep levels of antioxidants high in your body and you'll slow down the ageing process.

Lazy girl's version: your mum wasn't lying when she said those vegetables were good for you!

Aromatherapy

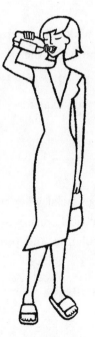

Technical version: the massaging in of various essential oils – about 400 of them in total – to help ease anxiety, stress and also treat problems such as spots and skin irritations.

Lazy girl's version: nice-smelling oils that look good in your bathroom.

Ayurvedic medicine

Technical version: Ayurveda, meaning 'the science of life', is a holistic method, which analyses a person's lifestyle as part of the treatment.

Lazy girl's version: trendy Indian alternative medicine, which is also sneaking its influence into the beauty arena.

Botox injections

Technical version: Botox gets rid of horizontal creases in the forehead and frown lines and involves a cosmetic surgeon injecting minute quantities of Botox into contracted muscles to help smooth them out.

Lazy girl's version: facial injections, which contain a strand of poison to paralyse your forehead muscles so you can look forever young (well, for three months anyway).

Cannula

Technical version: a thin, hollow tube, which is inserted into the skin during liposuction operations for the purpose of sucking out fat.

Lazy girl's version: the cosmetic-surgery equivalent of a vacuum nozzle.

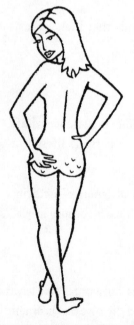

Cathiodermie facial

Technical version: a posher-than-average facial whereby rollers that carry minute amounts of electrical current are rolled across your skin to improve circulation and promote radiance.

Lazy girl's version: hardworking facial booster.

Cellulite

Technical version: deposits of fat collected under the skin, leading to a dimpled orange-peel look. Mainly the result of lifestyle choices, not genes, but can be lessened by improving your diet and including exercise and deep massage.

Lazy girl's version: squishy, dimpled skin on the thighs and bottom. The result of doing all the things you love to do but know you shouldn't.

Ceramides

Technical version: these work on a cell level and help the skin by supporting the structure and trapping moisture. They are usually found in creams for older women.

Lazy girl's version: more moisture for older, drier skins.

Chemical peel

Technical version: relatively severe beauty treatment that works by applying a chemical acid to your face to peel away the upper layers of skin, to leave you (eventually) with soft baby skin.

Lazy girl's version: the facial equivalent of peeling away the layers of an onion.

Collagen

Technical version: a natural part of human skin, which keeps your cheeks bouncy, fresh and plump-looking.

Without collagen the skin becomes saggy, crêpe-like and wrinkled.

Lazy girl's version: your natural skin firmer.

Colonic irrigation

Technical version: colonic irrigation is an assisted way of flushing out the bowel. Purified water is pumped through the colon via a tube to help flush out stored faecal matter and toxic substances.

Lazy girl's version: a procedure whereby a tube is pushed up your bottom and water poured in and flushed out.

Crystal clear

Technical version: a brand name for a dermabrasion technique beloved of celebrities, which works by blasting the skin with fine granules over six sessions.

Lazy girl's version: posh skin-sanding.

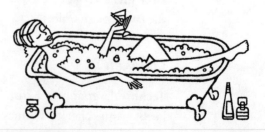

Dandruff

Technical version: an overgrowth of normal fungus found on the scalp. It causes the scales of dead skin to be shed from the scalp in small white bits.

Lazy girl's version: flaky scalp.

Deep vein thrombosis

Technical version: deep vein thrombosis is the formation of large blood clots in the leg. Under normal everyday conditions the movement of the calf muscle in the leg pumps blood back to the heart keeping the circulation in the body going. However, in situations where a person is immobile and/or cramped for a long period of time, such as on a plane, blood can pool and a clot can form in the leg; this clot can later travel to the heart and lungs with fatal consequences.

Lazy girl's version: avoid DVT by walking around and stretching your legs out at least once every half-hour when travelling on a long-haul flight.

Dermabrasion

Technical version: the resurfacing of the skin using something abrasive like fine crystals or some kind of device.

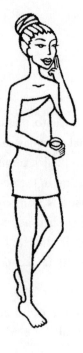

Lazy girl's version: sandblasting your skin to get a smoother surface.

Detox

Technical version: a spring-clean system where you eat basic food, such as rice and vegetables, and water in order to rid the body of harmful toxins, which give you dull skin and no energy.

Lazy girl's version: the fruit and vegetable diet that eliminates everything you like.

Eczema

Technical version: inflammatory skin disease that usually appears on the hands, inside the elbows and behind the knees. Treatment is by steroid creams from doctors, herbalism or homeopathy.

Lazy girl's version: dry, scaly, thickened skin, itching and redness, sometimes blisters.

Elastin

Technical version: this is the connective fibre, which supports the skin, giving it that bounce-back effect.

Lazy girl's version: the trampoline layer of your skin.

Endermologie

Technical version: a proven cellulite treatment that is basically a deep-tissue massage using a machine to pummel your cells back into shape.

Lazy girl's version: being pummelled by a hand-held machine.

Escin

Technical version: also known as horse chestnut tree extract – an active ingredient to help beat cellulite.

Lazy girl's version: alternative cellulite treatment.

Exfoliation

Technical version: products that allow you to scrub your skin so that you dislodge and slough off dead skin layers that leave your skin looking dull.

Lazy girl's version: a vigorous facial using a cream with hard bits in.

Free radicals

Technical version: molecules that destroy cells in the body and come in the form of pollution, smoking and too much of the party life. They contribute towards ageing so it's best to avoid them.

Lazy girl's version: environmental nasties – protect yourself by eating more fruit and vegetables.

Humectants

Technical version: an ingredient in moisturisers that works by attracting water droplets from the air, thereby keeping your skin moist.

Lazy girl's version: fancy term for a water magnet.

Keratin

Technical version: the protein that's found in hair and nails.

Lazy girl's version: one of the first proteins to lose their gusto when you live it up and don't look after your diet (think split ends and brittle nails).

Liposomes

Technical version: moisture- and nutrient-filled packs that travel deeper than most ingredients. Most contain vitamin E and anti-ageing retinol.

Lazy girl's version: something that may work in a skin cream

Liposuction

Technical version: liposuction is a cosmetic-surgery procedure whereby a tube is stuck into a small incision in the skin and fat tissue is literally vacuumed out. Usually used on inner thighs, bottoms, chins and stomachs.

Lazy girl's version: think of a vacuum sucking fat out of your body ...

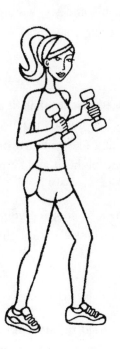

Pilates

Technical version: a mind-body exercise regime that's akin to a yoga. It's based on building a strong core group of muscles, body realignment and resistance work.

Lazy girl's version: lean, stretching, postural exercise.

Reflexology

Technical version: this is the practice of applying pressure to points on the feet and hands, which correspond to areas of the body, to stimulate the body's own healing system.

Lazy girl's version: a deep foot massage.

Retinol

Technical version: a new anti-ageing ingredient that comes from vitamin A. It's not the same as Retin-A, which is a prescription drug that can be given only by your doctor.

Lazy girl's version: yet another use-this and stay young for ever cream.

Rosacea

Technical version: Rosacea, pronounced rose-ay-shah, is a disease affecting the skin and causing red flushed patches on the face. It usually starts off looking like sunburn or acne but can spread along the cheeks, forehead and chin making the face look very red.

Lazy girl's version: control the redness by spotting your triggers: alcohol, chocolate, spicy foods, stress, sunlight and extreme temperatures can all make it worse.

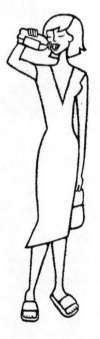

Silicone

Technical version: not the stuff once used in boob jobs, but a ingredient now found in many hair products as it adds shine and sleekness to hair. Most hair serums that promise anti-frizz qualities contain silicone. Also used as a filler on facial lines.

Lazy girl's version: the stuff that makes your hair go limp and lumpy, if you use too much of it.

Sunblock

Technical version: a chemical-based cream that acts as a barrier against the sun's UVA and UVB rays.

Lazy girl's version: the cream that will stop you looking like an aged prune.

UVA/UVB rays

Technical version: ultraviolet rays. UVB are the rays that burn your skin and UVA rays are the ones that speed up the ageing process and cause skin cancer. In order to protect yourself you need a sunscreen that offers protection from both.

Lazy girl's version: if you can only manage to do one beauty-related thing, make sure you wear sunscreen with a sun protection factor (SPF) of at least 15.

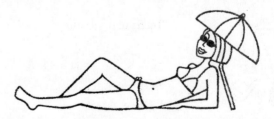

Vitamins

Technical version: naturally occurring substances that are essential for a healthy body and life. The best way to get them is through your food intake because this aids their integration into the body and helps them to work effectively.

Lazy girl's version: all the nutrients you avoid if you stick to a low-calorie or junk- and alcohol-based diet.

Zzzz ... sleep

Technical version: sleep is our natural state of rest and is essential if you want to be beautiful and happy. Aim for between seven and nine hours a night.

Lazy girl's version: there's a reason why they call it beauty sleep!

Resources

UK

Association of Personal Trainers
PO Box 6131, London SW9 9XR
Tel: 020 8692 4023

Balance (colonic hydrotherapy)
250 Kings Road, London SW3 5UE
Tel: 020 7565 0333

British Acupuncture Council
63 Jeddo Road, London W12 9HQ
Tel: 020 8735 0400 Website: www.acupuncture.org.uk

Beauty on the net
www.hqhair.com – hair advice and hair products
www.wellbeing.com – information, and products from
Boots

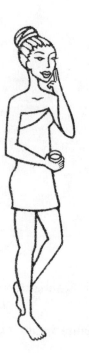

www.emakemeup.com – advice from make-up artists
www.beautyriot.com – celebrity looks
www.pout.co.uk – glitzy and gorgeous make-up products

British Association of Aesthetic Plastic Surgeons
Website: www.baaps.co.uk

British Complementary Medicine Association
Tel: 0845 345 5977

British Dental Association (to find a dentist)
Website: www.bda-dentistry.org.uk

British Osteopathic Association
Tel: 01582 488455 Website: www.osteopathy.org.uk

BUPA (plastic surgery)
Tel: 0845 600 8822 Website: www.bupahospitals.co.uk

Care Standards Commission (plastic surgery)
Website: www.carestandards.org.uk

Fellowship of Sports Masseurs and Therapists
PO Box 81, Hertford, SG13 7WJ
Tel: 01992 537778

Indian Head Massage
Website: www.indianchampissage.com

Massage
For a round-up of all the massage therapies available in
the UK and practitioners in your area
Website: www.massagetherapy.co.uk

Shiatsu
Website: info@londoncollegeofshiatsu.com

Sleep Council
Tel: 0800 018 7923 Website: www.sleepcouncil.org.uk

Society of Chiropodists
54 Station Road, London NW10 4UA
Tel: 020 8961 4006

Spas in the UK
Healthy Venues, for unbiased advice and brochures from
UK spas and health farms
Tel: 0870 850 5550 Website: www.healthyvenues.co.uk

Stress (for information and links to stress organisations)
Website: www.stress.org.uk

Stress Management
Tel: 020 8293 4114 Website: www.managingstress.com

Thai Massage
Website: www.thaitherapy.com

The Pilates Foundation (for a trained teacher in your area) Tel: 07071 781859 Website: www.pilatesfoundation.com or www.bodycontrol.co.uk

Yoga links
www.bikramyoga.com – Bikram Yoga
www.triyoga.com – Triyoga - London
www.iyi.org.uk – Iyengar yoga
www.bwy.org.uk – British Wheel of Yoga
www.sivananda.org – Sivananda yoga

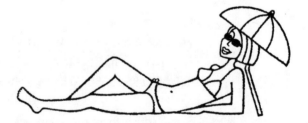

Australia

International yoga teachers
Website: www.iyta.org.au

Pilates Institute of Australasia
Website: www.pilates.net

Plastic Surgery
Website: www.asps.asn.au

Spas
Websites:
www.aurorasparetreat.com
and www.daintree-ecolodge.co.au
Aveda day Spa www.asabu.com.au

New Zealand

Pilates
Website: www.clinicalpilates.com/nz

Plastic Surgery
Website: www.nzdoctor.co.nz/links.htm

Spas
Websites: www.polynesianspa.co.nz
and www.taupohotsprings.com

Yoga Academy
Website: www.yoga.co.nz

South Africa

Pilates
Website: www.bodycontrol.co.uk/south.africa.html

Plastic Surgery
Website: www.plasticsurgeons.co.za/home.htm

Spas
Websites: www.fancourt.co.za and www.serenite.co.za

Yoga
Website: www.yoga.com

index